Clinical Tests
Ophthalmology

M.J.E. Huber
MRCP FRCS
Visiting Associate Professor
Sultan Qaboos University
Muscat, Oman

M.H. Reacher
FRCS FCOphth MPH
Fellow, Wilmer Institute
Johns Hopkins University
Baltimore, Maryland, USA

Wolfe Medical Publications Ltd

Copyright © M.J.E. Huber, M.H. Reacher, 1990
First published 1990 by Wolfe Medical Publications Ltd
Printed by W.S. Cowell Ltd, Ipswich, England
ISBN 0 7234 0976 5
ISSN 0952 6986

No part of this publication may be reproduced, copied or transmitted save with written permission or in accordance with the provisions of the Copyright Act 1956 (as amended), or under the terms of any licence permitting limited copying issued by the Copyright Licensing Agency, 33-34 Alfred Place, London, WC1E 7DP.

Any person who does any unauthorised act in relation to this publication may be liable to criminal prosecution and civil claims for damages.

A CIP catalogue record for this book is available from the British Library.

This book is one of the titles in the series of Wolfe Medical Atlases, a series which brings together probably the world's largest systematic published collection of diagnostic colour photographs.

For a full list of atlases in the series, plus forthcoming titles and details of our surgical, dental and veterinary atlases, please write to Wolfe Medical Publications Ltd, 2-16 Torrington Place, London WC1E 7LT, England.

Contents

Acknowledgements	4
1. Introduction	5
2. Testing visual acuity	6
3. Examining infants and children	15
4. Neuro-ophthalmology	16
5. Tests for squint	53
6. Tests of lacrimal function	64
7. Use of the slit-lamp	72
8. Tests relevant to the conjunctiva, cornea and anterior chamber	79
9. Tests in glaucoma	91
10. Tests for posterior segment diagnosis	118
11. Tests in ocular injuries	141
12. Basic tests in optics	145
13. Tests for systemic disease	165
References	170
Index	174

Acknowledgements

We are most grateful to the patients and our friends and colleagues from St. Thomas' Hospital, Greenwich District Hospital, Moorfields Eye Hospital and Queen Elizabeth Military Hospital, London, England and The Wilmer Institute, Johns Hopkins Hospital, Baltimore, USA for their help in preparing the illustrations for this book.

We would also like to thank the following for kindly letting us use their slides:

Dr J Bingham **69**; Mr J Chesterton **66, 67**; Dr S DeBoustros **211**;
Mr R Dewhurst **202, 203**; Mr T George **113, 129, 130, 131**;
Dr J Gottsch **117, 118, 121**; Dr E Graham **204, 205**; Dr N Iliff **213**;
Dr M Johnson **70, 71, 73, 74, 75**; Dr N Miller **49, 50, 51, 161, 162**;
Dr H Quigley **160**; Dr M Restori **196, 197, 198, 199**; Dr N Sandhu **68**;
Mr J Shilling **208, 209, 210, 212**; Mr D Spalton **43, 44**; Dr H Taylor **123, 124**; Dr S West **115**.

1 Introduction

Ophthalmology differs from general medicine in that the basic examination of patients requires complex instruments, the use of which will be described here. It is insufficient merely to describe ophthalmic signs, they must be quantified as far as possible so that improvement or deterioration can be monitored, and methods of doing this with particular signs are included. All findings, both normal and abnormal, should be clearly documented for both eyes—unilateral conditions may become bilateral and a written record of previously normal status is essential.

The examination of a new patient should always include the best corrected visual acuity in each eye, the presence or absence of a relative afferent pupil defect and tonometry in all patients over 40 years of age (and younger where relevant). A thorough evaluation should include:

History: ophthalmic, general medical, drugs, allergies and family.

Examination:
    At the desk: *ocular function*
        visual acuity (best corrected), distance and reading
        colour vision
        visual field test to confrontation
        swinging flashlight test
        eye movements
    At the slit-lamp: *anterior segment and intra-ocular pressure*
        lids
        conjunctiva
        cornea
        anterior chamber and iris
        applanation tonometry
    After dilatation: *the lens and posterior segment*
        lens
        vitreous
        fundus (including disc and macula)

Further examination and investigations as indicated.

2 Testing visual acuity

Infants and children

The human face is the best target for fixation and following in the neonate.

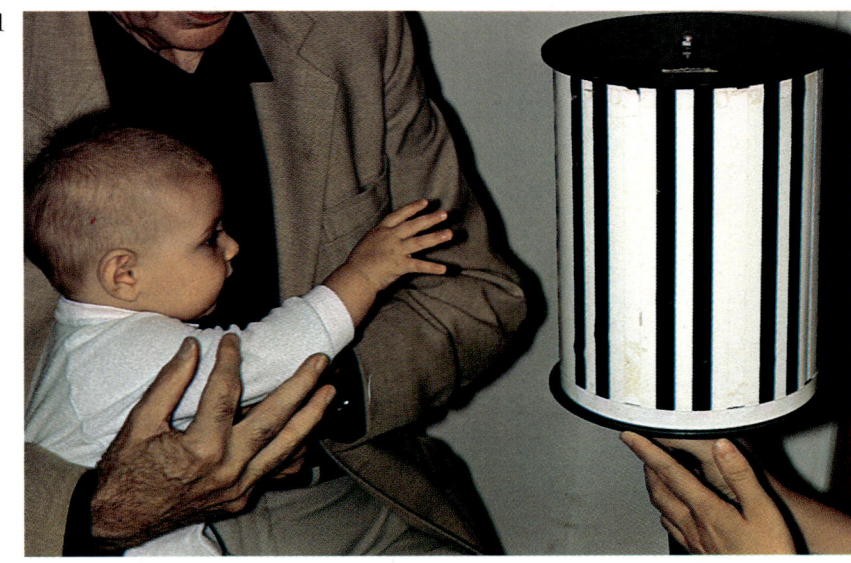

1 Optokinetic nystagmus. The drum is rotated slowly. The child's eyes move to follow one stripe then jerk back to watch the next stripe. The Catford drum uses round targets which move back and forth. For each test the resultant eye movements are observed.

2 Objecting to occlusion. Infants usually object to occlusion of an eye with good vision. The passive acceptance of occlusion suggests the vision is poor in the occluded eye.

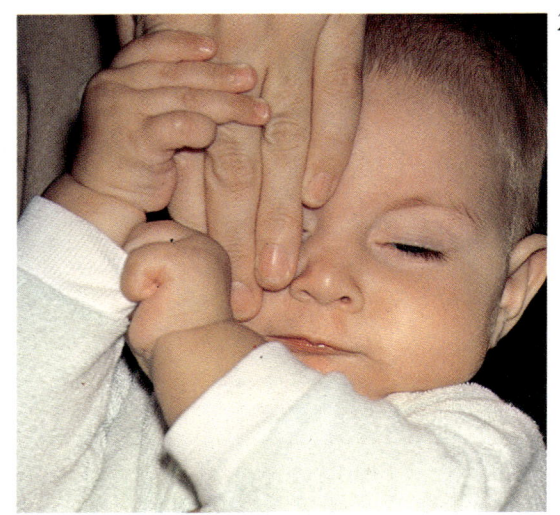

3 Picking up tiny objects. These will be picked up accurately between thumb and finger by infants of nine months or older where sight is normal, or will be fumbled for where they are poorly seen. Significant refractive errors do not, however, greatly diminish the ability to see and pick up tiny objects.

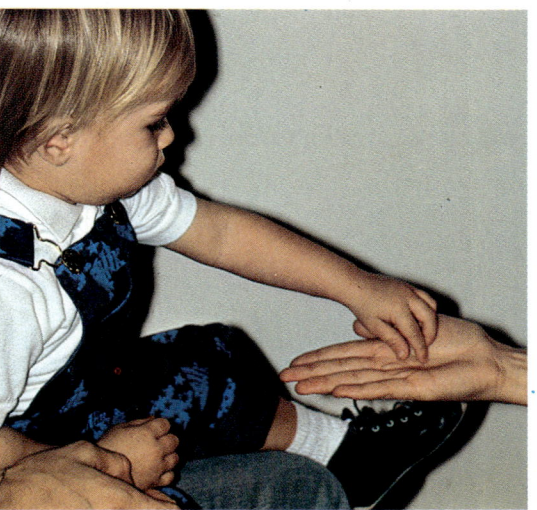

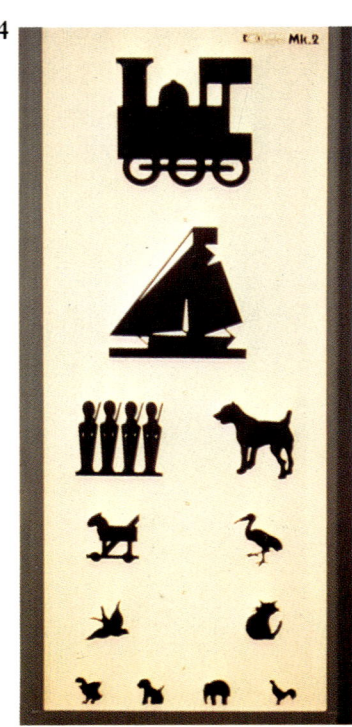

4 Symbol chart. Children of 2 to 3 years can recognize symbols but initially the chart may need to be explained when held close up to the child.

5 Sheridan Gardiner matching letter test. A child of 3 years old or over can look at a letter in the distance and select a matching letter from the card. A multiple optotype chart (**6**) is used in preference to single optotypes because amblyopes may have a better acuity when reading single letters than when reading a line of letters.

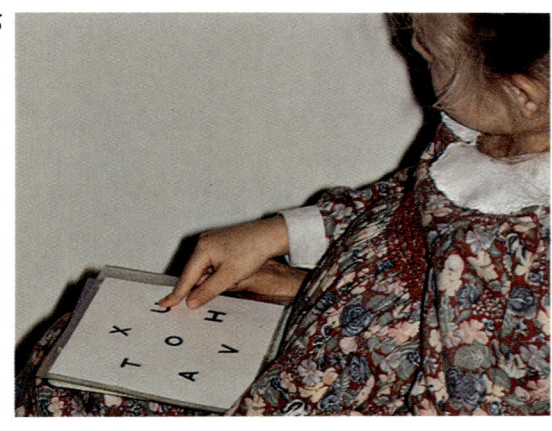

Adults

In order to distinguish refractive error from ocular pathology it is essential to know the corrected visual acuity of a patient. Distance vision and near (reading) vision are tested separately. Both must be tested because in some conditions, e.g. high myopia or cataracts, the patient may only see 'counting fingers' for distance but see N5 for near and so have functionally effective vision.

6 Test chart. Letters subtending different angles at the macula are used. Visual acuity measured with test charts is diminished by reduced contrast caused by poor illumination. The chart should be bright and the room well lit. In most clinical settings, exact standardization of illumination is not observed.

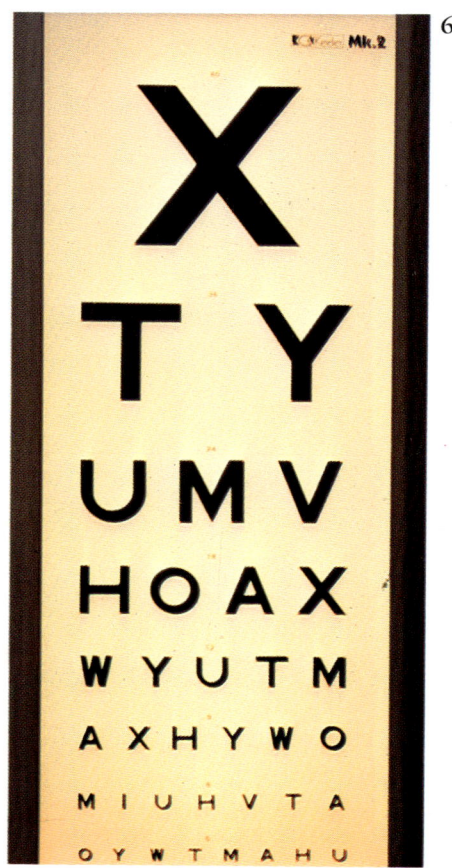

6

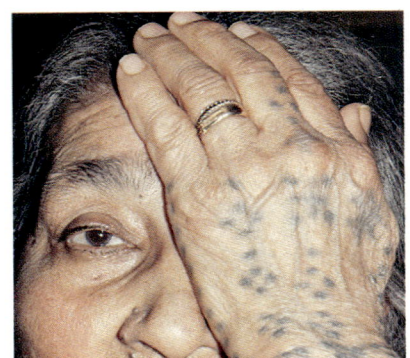

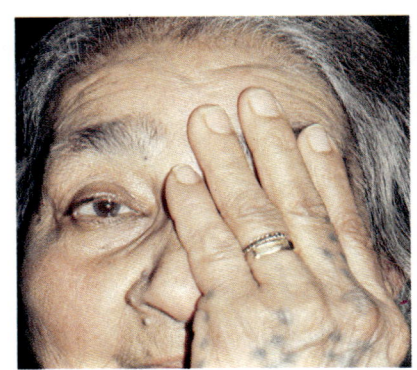

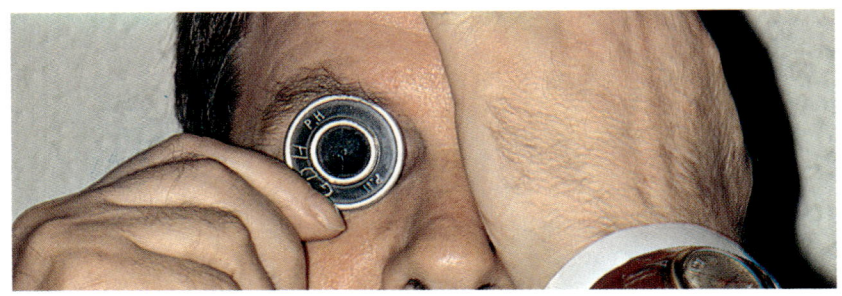

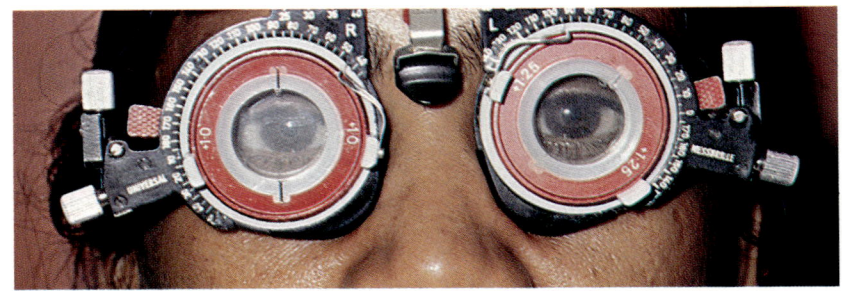

7 Occluding the eye. The eyes are tested separately, right first. The other eye must be firmly covered with the palm of the hand or an occluder.

8 Incorrect occlusion. The patient should not use her fingers to cover the other eye or she may look between them.

9 Pinhole correction. A pinhole (stenopaeic aperture) will compensate for many refractive errors. It may worsen the vision in corneal or vitreous opacities, but improve it in cataract.

10 Refraction. Reliable best visual acuity requires refraction and appropriate lens correction (see Chapter 12).

If the vision is less than 6/60 (20/200) the patient is brought nearer the chart and the notation altered accordingly e.g. 3/60 (20/400). The first number in the Snellen notation is the distance at which the test is performed (6 metres or 20 feet), the second number relates to the size of the test letter.

11 Vision of 1/60 (20/1200) or less. Vision of 1/60 roughly corresponds to 'counting fingers' vision, i.e. the patient can correctly count the number of fingers shown at 1 m. It may be necessary to hold the fingers nearer the patient's face. If fingers cannot be counted accurately on several attempts the hand should be moved in front of the eye to detect 'hand movement' perception.

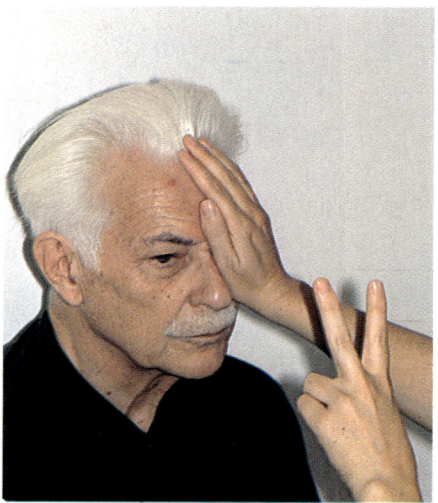

12 Vision less than 'hand movements'. If the patient cannot see hand movements, light perception is tested with a bright light. Patients should state whether the light is on or not, but they may guess the answer, therefore the test must be repeated several times, with and without the light shining to check their accuracy. If light perception exists, the function of different parts of the retina is tested by directing the light at the eye from each of the four quadrants and asking the patient to point at it ('light projection').

13 E chart. Illiterates or patients who use a different alphabet to the available test chart are shown an E and asked to point in the direction of the prongs of the E.

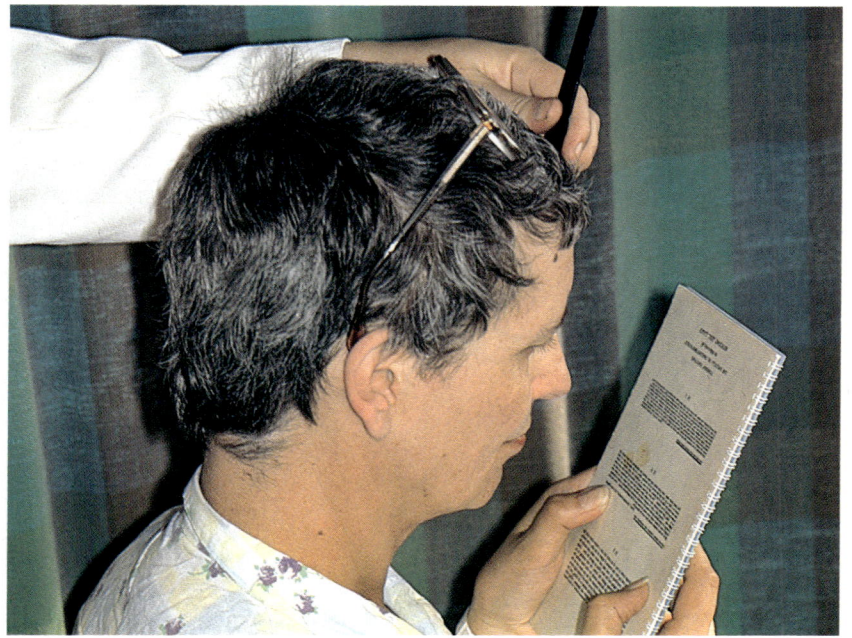

14 Near (reading) vision. Patients with an acuity of counting fingers or more are examined using a near reading chart at a standard distance of 30 cm (or if a chart is unavailable the small print in a newspaper is used). Each eye should be tested separately. Presbyopic patients require a reading correction for a meaningful result. Some patients, e.g. high myopes, may need to remove their glasses and hold the chart very close to their faces to read, as illustrated, and should be shown how to do this. However, this does not provide a true index of acuity because the letters now subtend a larger angle at the eye.

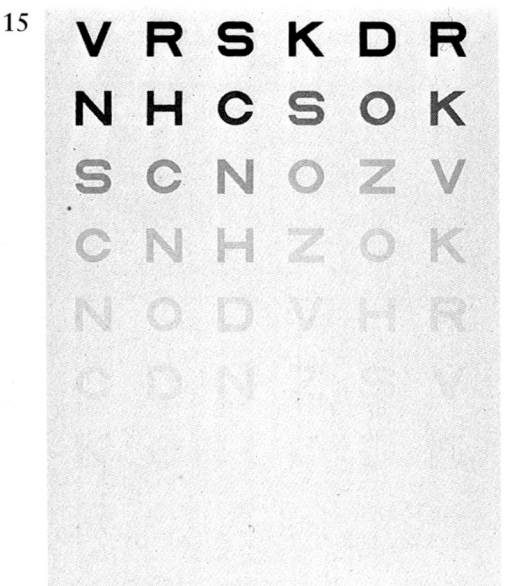

15 Contrast sensitivity. Afferent visual function can also be measured by assessing the patient's ability to detect differences in contrast. This may be tested with the Pelli-Robson Letter Sensitivity Chart (Copyright © 1988 Denis G. Pelli) shown here, in which letters decrease in contrast, not in size. This is a more sensitive indicator of function than Snellen acuity, and may provide earlier detection of retinal and optic nerve disease.

3 Examining infants and children

As much as possible should be observed while a baby is asleep or not crying. Visual acuity should be tested even at a young age (see Chapter 2). Pupil examination provides indirect information about vision and is combined with anterior segment examination. Infants can be held up to the slit-lamp.

Tonometry, gonioscopy, and examination for suspected ocular trauma require sedation or a general anaesthetic in the very young, though examination of the fundi and retinoscopy through dilated pupils are usually possible without anaesthetic. Most anaesthetic agents decrease intra-ocular pressure, apart from ketamine which slightly increases it. Therefore ketamine may be the agent of choice. Tonometry is performed immediately after induction. Premedication, except for systemic atropine, should be avoided (see also Chapter 5).

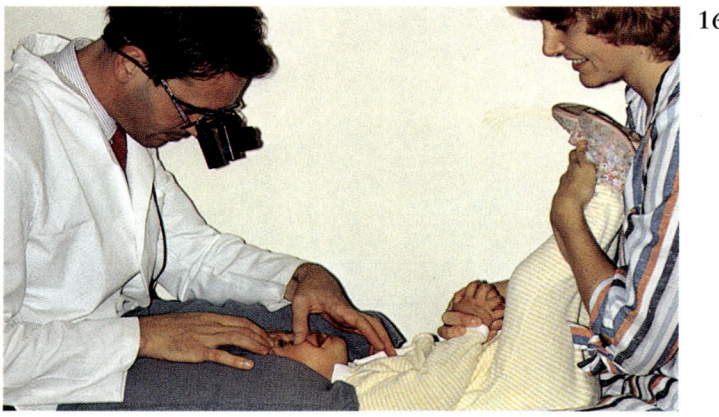

16

16 Infant restraint. This may be achieved by the relative holding the infant while the examiner holds the head between his knees. The lids are opened without pressure on the globe by skin traction over the orbital margins, or Desmarres lid retractors are inserted beneath upper then lower lids to lift them off the globe. Once a penetrating injury has been excluded, upper lid eversion is performed. A binocular loupe with illumination is a considerable asset. This technique is suitable for primary eye care.

4 Neuro-ophthalmology

Unless a basic neuro-ophthalmological evaluation is included in the examination of new patients (see Chapter 1), the examiner will one day miss a pituitary tumour or a nutritional optic neuropathy.

Colour vision

This can be tested by relying entirely on the patient's impression or by using external criteria e.g. pseudo-ischromatic test plates (**18-21**). Ideally, both tests are performed as there may be considerable loss of colour vision before abnormal results are seen with test plates. More extensive tests to evaluate colour vision are available (e.g. the Farnsworth-Munsell 100 Hue Test) but these are more time consuming. Red-green colour vision is a sensitive indicator of optic nerve function.

17 Colour vision. The worse eye is occluded. The patient looks at a red target with the better eye (e.g. the right) and notes the colour, e.g. 'bright red', or the brightness is subjectively scored out of 10. The better eye is then occluded. The patient looks at the target with the worse eye (e.g. the left) and notes the colour relative to the better eye e.g. 'Dim red' or '5 out of 10' would indicate red desaturation typical of a left optic nerve lesion.

The red target should be uniformly lit, preferably by daylight. Answers such as 'the outline is blurred on the left' or 'bits of the pin are missing' do not mean the colour is abnormal. These answers may be given with refractive errors or pathology of the central retina or media. The patient must be specifically questioned about the colour and may reply that the target looks pink, black, pale, etc.

18 Ishihara test plates. These are commonly available and though originally designed for detecting congenital red-green colour vision deficiency (protanopia, deuteranopia), they are also used to test for acquired abnormalities of red-green vision. (Depending on the population examined, between 2 and 8 per cent of males have x-linked red-green colour blindness.) The congenitally colour deficient person makes standard predictable errors and misreadings listed in the explanation of the plates provided with them. Those with optic nerve disease find all the plates, except the first, more difficult and their errors are unpredictable.

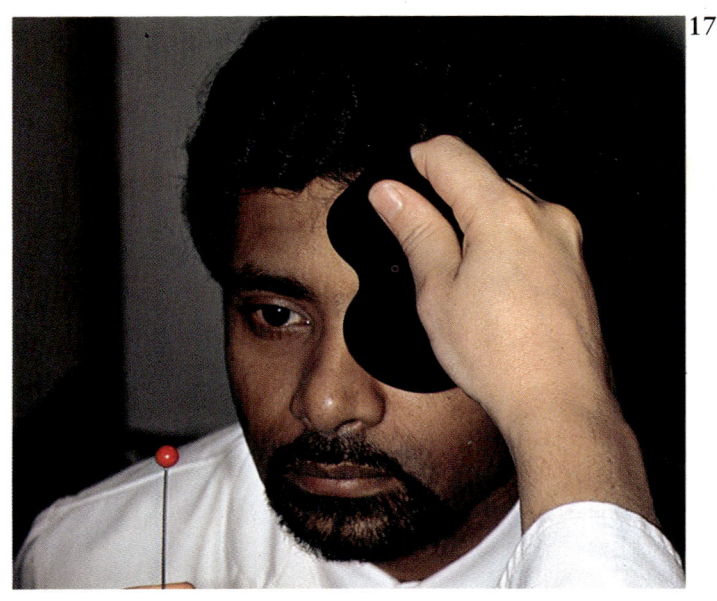

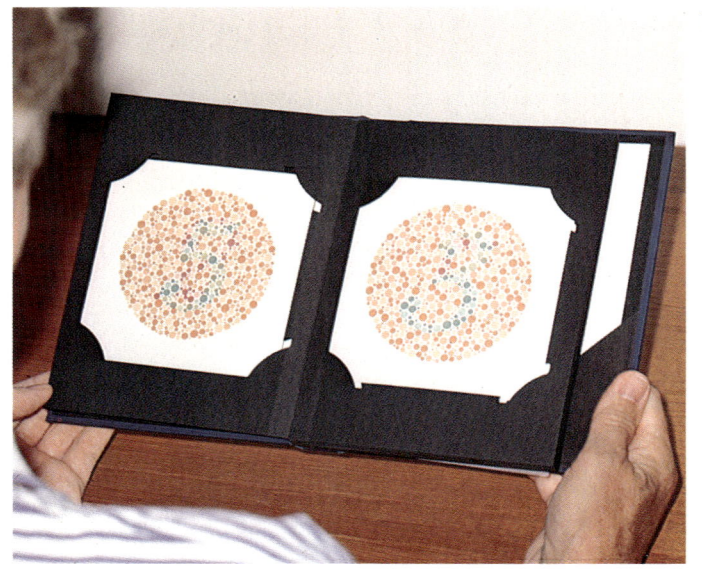

These plates are not designed to test blue-yellow colour deficiencies. The congenital ones (tritanopia, tritanomaly) are rare. In the acquired ones (macular disease) colour vision is a less important diagnostic point than in optic nerve disease.

19

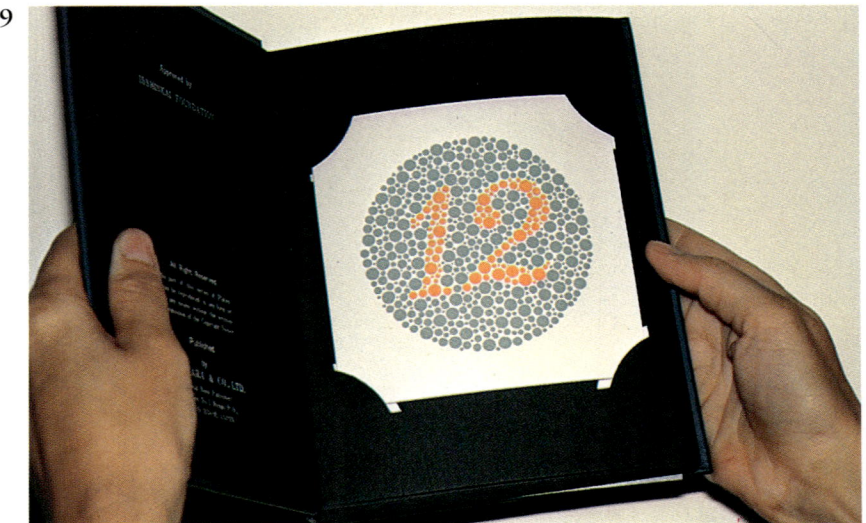

19 The contrast plate. Plate no. 1 has a difference in contrast between the number and the background, as well as a difference in colour. A patient with poor colour vision should still be able to read it unless his acuity is grossly impaired. Malingerers may deny being able to read the number.

20 Reading the plates. Test in diffuse daylight if possible. In suspected optic nerve disease plates 1 to 13 are read with each eye separately and the results recorded out of 13, e.g. right eye: 8/13 (contrast plate seen). The patient should wear glasses if a refractive error or presbyopia exists. He may be able to trace the outline of the coloured numbers even if he cannot decipher them—this indicates that the colour vision is intact even though the acuity may be impaired for other reasons.

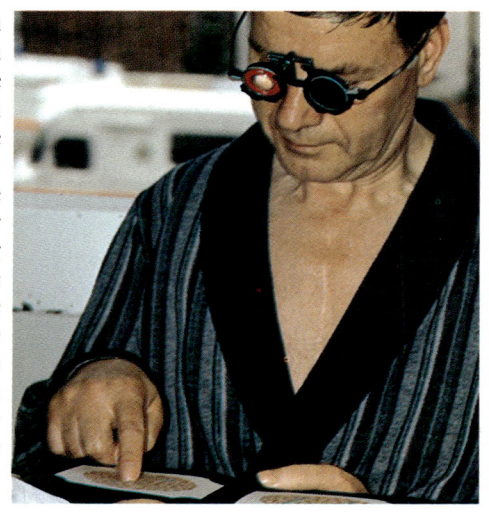

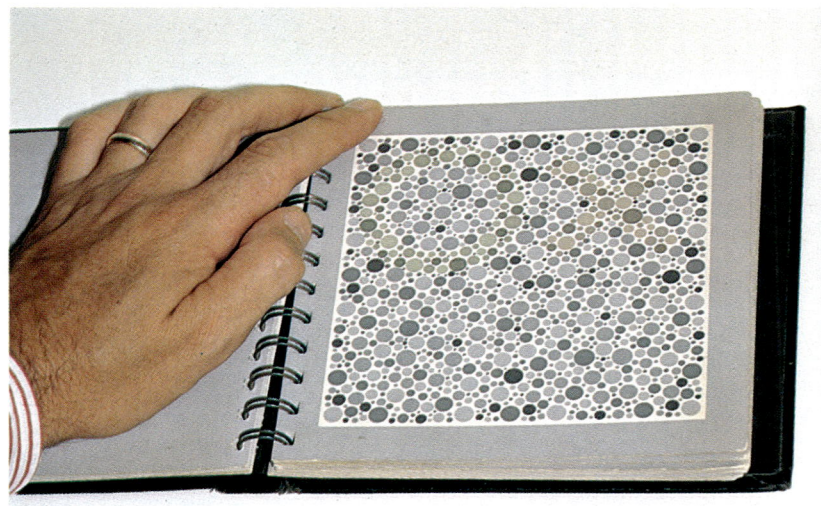

21 Hardy-Rand-Rittler test plates. These plates may be used to test for blue-yellow colour deficiencies in addition to red-green deficiencies.

Visual fields to confrontation

This test should be performed with the likely possible defects in mind, i.e. central scotomas, altitudinal field defects, and hemianopias (both homonymous and bitemporal). They are most sensitively detected with a small red target e.g. an 8 mm red pinhead or the red top of a mydriatic bottle.

The examiner must sit level with and facing the patient. One of the patient's eyes is occluded and the examiner shuts his own eye on the same side (e.g. the patient's left, the examiner's right eye). The patient is asked to look at the examiner's open eye, *not* at the moving target, and may need reminding of this during the test.

22 Testing the field to red. The target is shown centrally. If it is not seen, or is seen but the colour is desaturated, a central scotoma may be present. If this occurs, the target is moved outwards from the centre until it is fully seen with a normal bright red colour. This is done in several directions to delineate the scotoma.

23 Testing the field to red. The target is then brought in from the periphery, in all four quadrants, while the patient is reminded to look straight ahead. The patient is asked when he becomes aware of the red colour of the target. The examiner compares the patient's field to his own. Examining on either side of the vertical meridian will identify upper temporal loss in a chiasmal lesion.

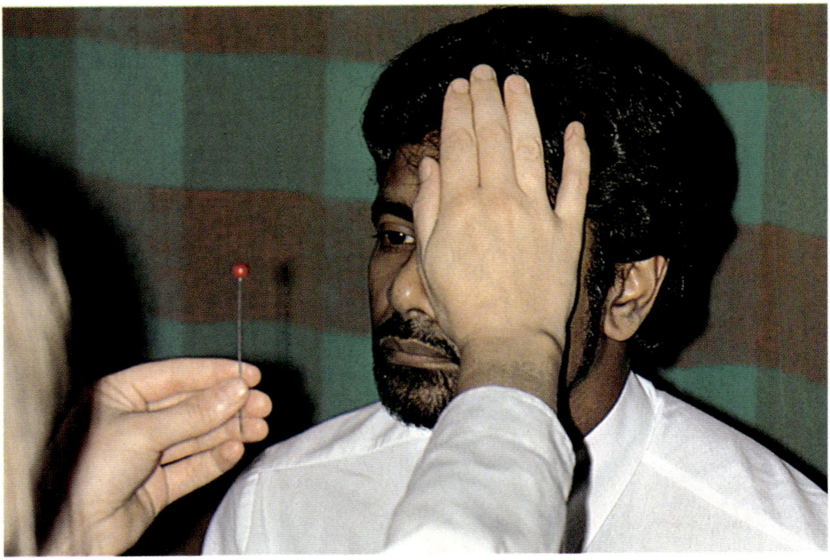

22

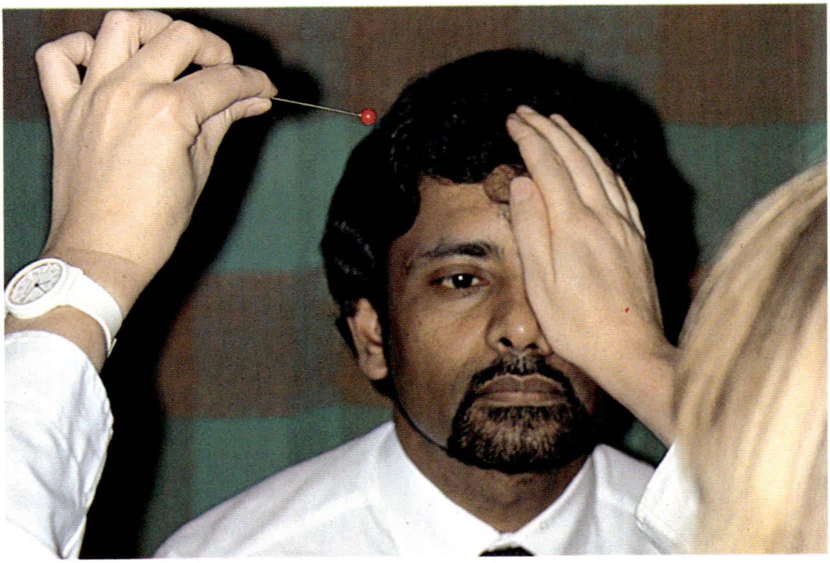

23

21

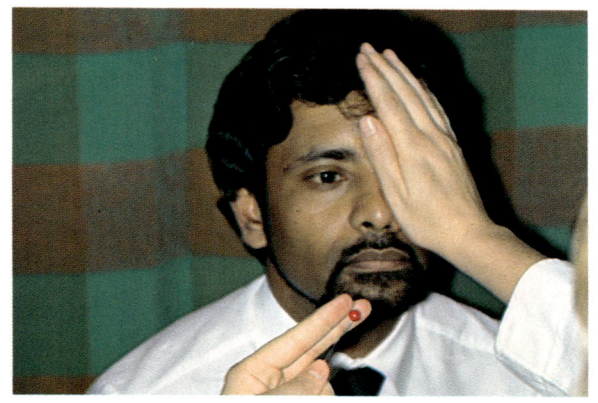

24 Checking that colour is being identified. The examiner may cover the target intermittently with his fingers to be sure that the patient is identifying the red colour and not the movement of the hand.

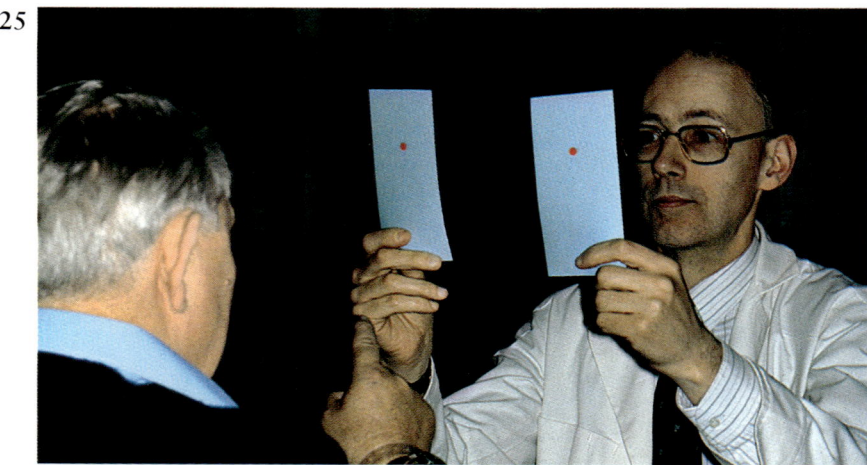

25 Comparing two targets. In a hemianopia (or altitudinal defect) a target held on one side of the vertical (or horizontal) meridian will be noticeably dimmer than a similar target held on the other side. The targets here are red dots on blue cards. The patient can indicate the dim side by pointing. The examiner's hands can also be used as targets for brightness comparison.

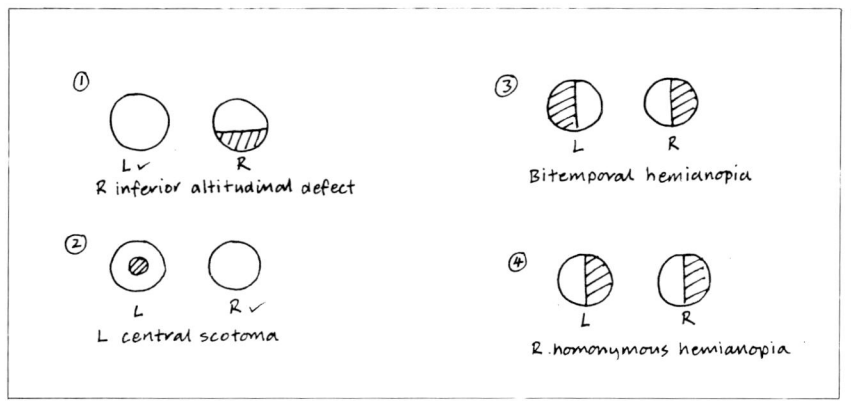

26 Recording results. By convention the results are recorded the way the patient sees them. These are common field defects as they might be recorded in the notes.

Formal visual field testing is required if a neuro-ophthalmological diagnosis is made (see Chapter 9).

Pupils: the swinging flashlight test

Observing the pupil sizes, the direct and consensual reactions to light and the reaction to accommodation and convergence, comprise a standard part of the examination. It is also essential to perform the swinging flashlight test, which demonstrates a relative afferent pupillary defect (RAPD). When illuminating the abnormal eye, immediately following the illumination of its relatively normal fellow, a relative impairment of pupil constriction is observed. It provides evidence of an optic nerve lesion or extensive retinal damage e.g. a total retinal detachment. Small retinal abnormalities such as macular lesions usually do not produce an RAPD nor do medial opacities, e.g. cataract or vitreous haemorrhage. An RAPD may be found without a clinically detectable afferent defect, for example an episode of retrobulbar neuritis may resolve to normal vision and brisk pupil reactions but still show an RAPD. Note that a unilateral visual defect does not produce assymmetry of pupil size.

The test must be performed with a bright flashlight in a dim room. The patient should fix a distant target to eliminate the accommodation/convergence response and the light is shone from below the eyes. Although attention is directed at the illuminated pupil, both pupils behave synchronously and are the same size due to the consensual light reflex throughout the test.

27 Right RAPD. The light is shone on the normal left eye (arrow). Both pupils constrict, the left directly, the right consensually.

28 Right RAPD. The light is then swung towards the defective right eye. Both pupils begin to dilate as the light crosses the bridge of the nose (arrow).

29 Right RAPD. As the light reaches the right eye (arrow), the pupils continue to dilate.

30 Right RAPD. On swinging back to the left eye (arrow), both pupils constrict. This sequence becomes more apparent as the torch is swung back and forth several times, pausing on each pupil.

27

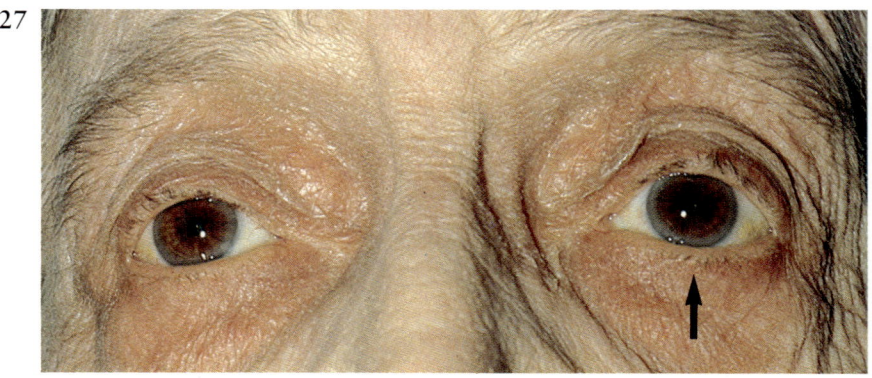

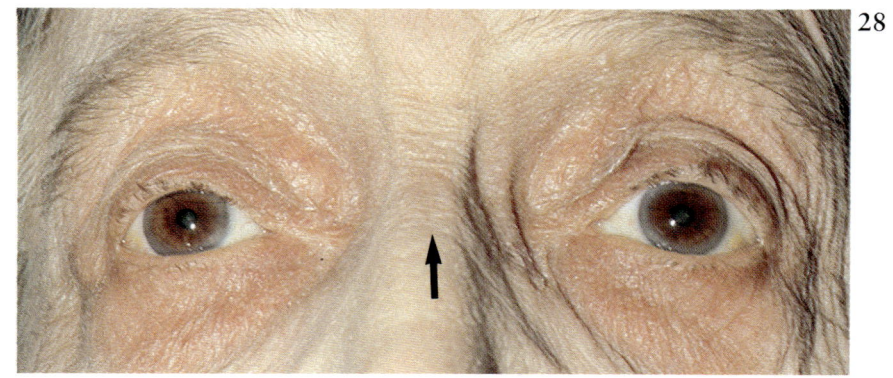

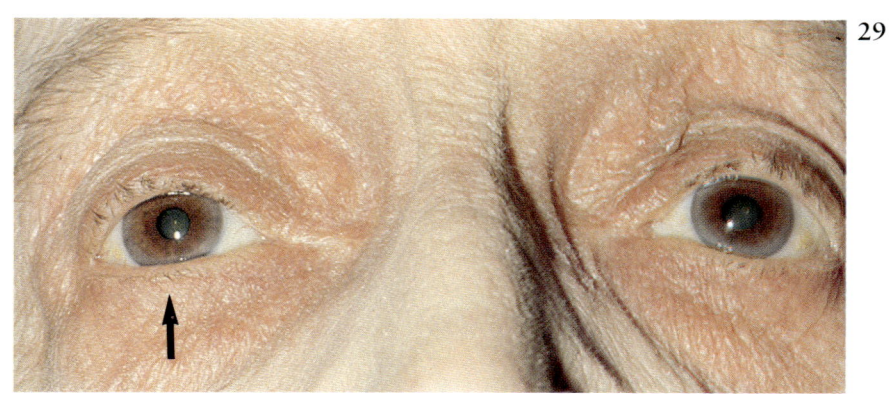

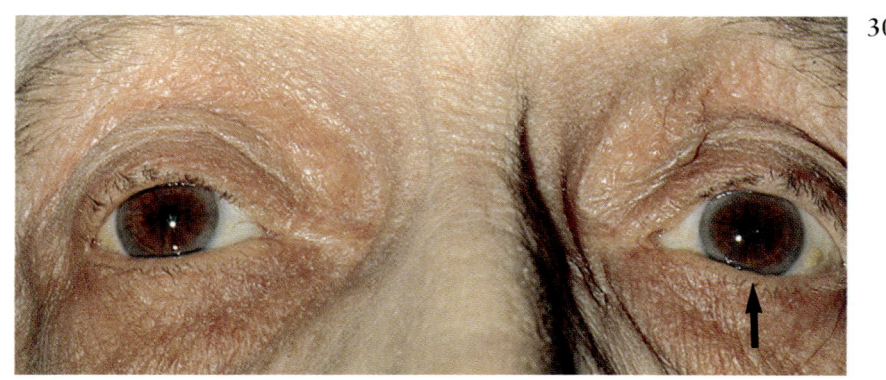

Eye movements

Infranuclear disorders
An awareness of the patterns of infranuclear disorders of eye movement is required to analyse them with ease (**42, 43, 45, 46**). The relevant muscle and nerve combinations are as follows:

	Dextroelevation		Levoelevation		
	RSR	III	LSR	III	
	LIO	III	RIO	III	
Dextroversion	RLR	VI	LLR	VI	Levoversion
	LMR	III	RMR	III	
	RIR	III	LIR	III	
	LSO	IV	RSO	IV	
	Dextrodepression		Levodepression		

The obliques reach the globe from the antero-medial aspect and so are aligned to elevate and depress when the eye is directed medially.

31 The primary position. The examiner inspects the eyes in the primary position as shown. Some defects will immediately be obvious, e.g. the ptosis and deviation of a complete IIIrd nerve palsy. The positions of the light reflexes on the corneas are compared. Asymmetry indicates a deviation.

The patient is asked to follow the target to the six diagnostic cardinal positions of gaze, dextroversion, dextroelevation and dextrodepression, and levoversion, levoelevation and levodepression, while keeping his head straight so that only his eyes move.

32 Dextroversion.

33 Dextroelevation.

34 Dextrodepression.

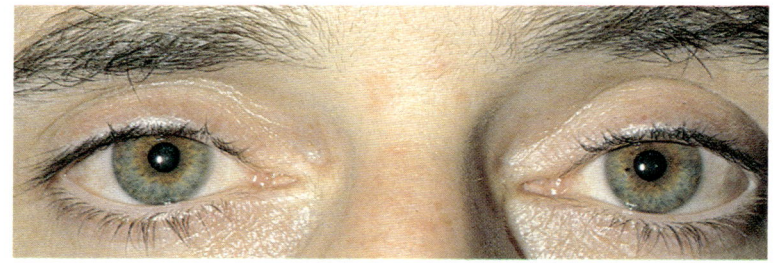

31

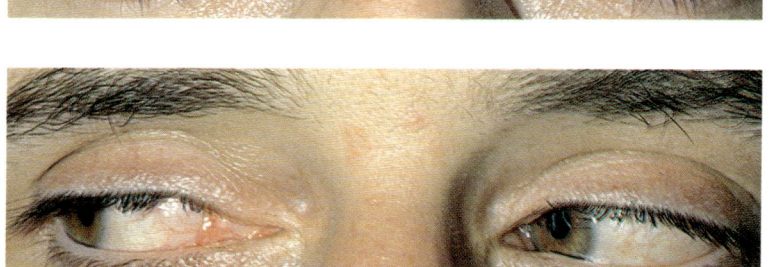

32

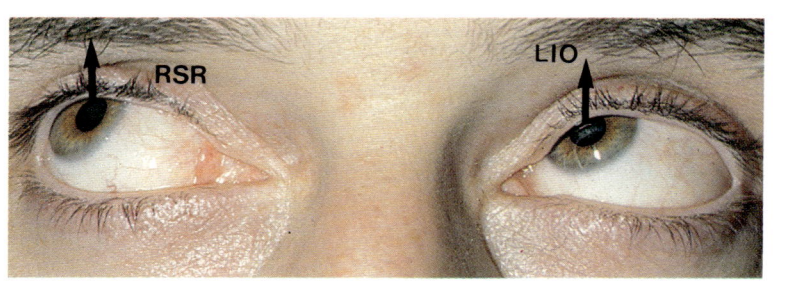

33

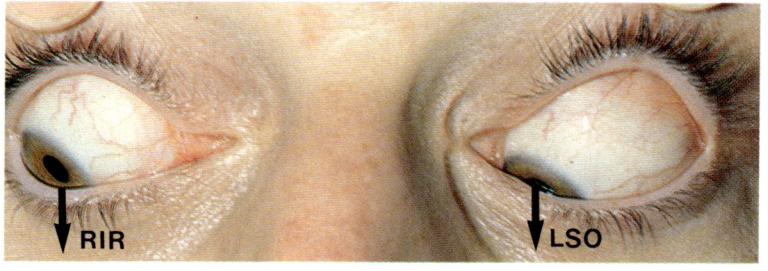

34

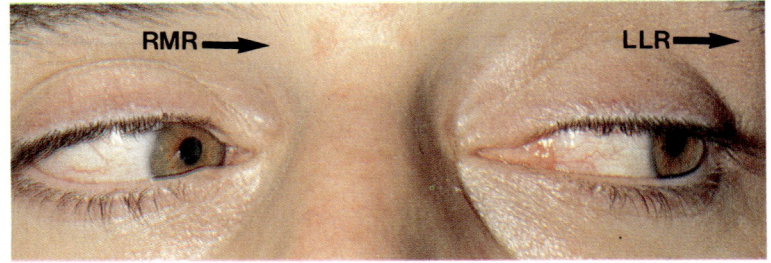

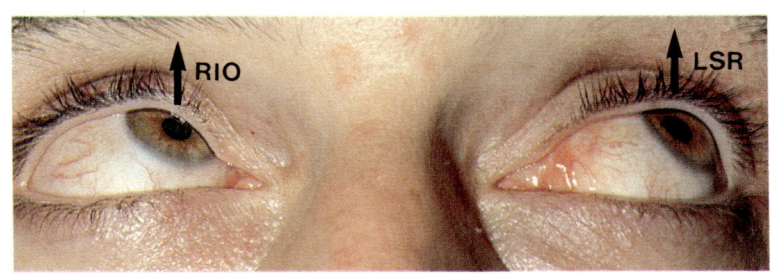

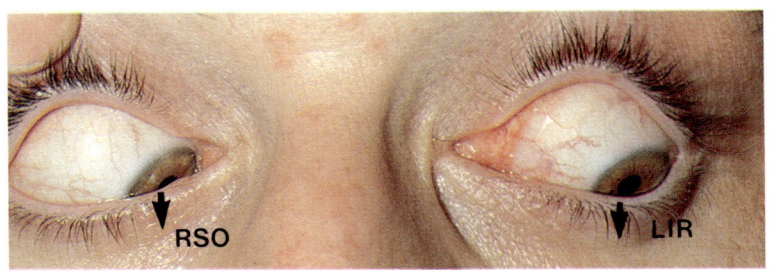

35 Levoversion.

36 Levoelevation.

37 Levodepression.

When performed in the central axis, elevation and depression involve the vertical recti and the obliques together and so are less helpful in elucidating single muscle and nerve problems. They assist in diagnosing orbital disorders and gaze pareses (e.g. failure of upward gaze in Parinaud's syndrome), and eliciting A and V phenomena in squint assessment.

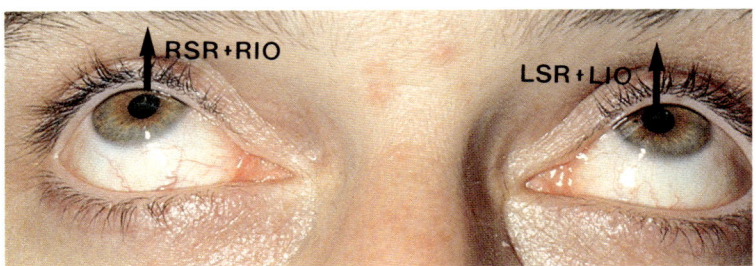

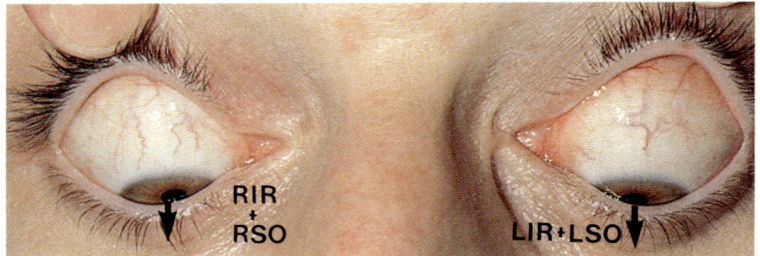

38 Elevation.

39 Depression.

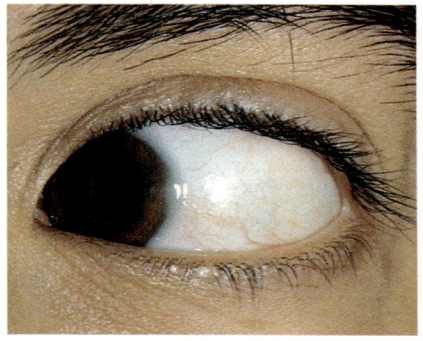 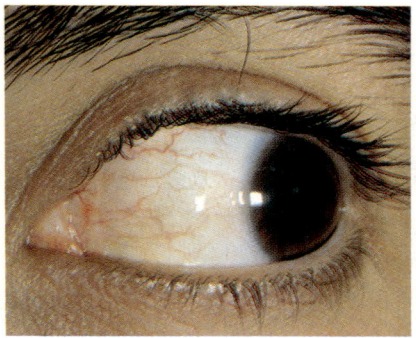

40 Extremes of gaze. The movement must be to the extremes of gaze as subtle defects may otherwise not be seen, and the observer must watch closely with the possible defects in mind. An adducting eye may bury 1 to 2 mm of the nasal cornea in the conjunctiva and caruncle.

41 Extremes of gaze. In an abducting eye the lateral cornea should virtually reach the outer canthus.

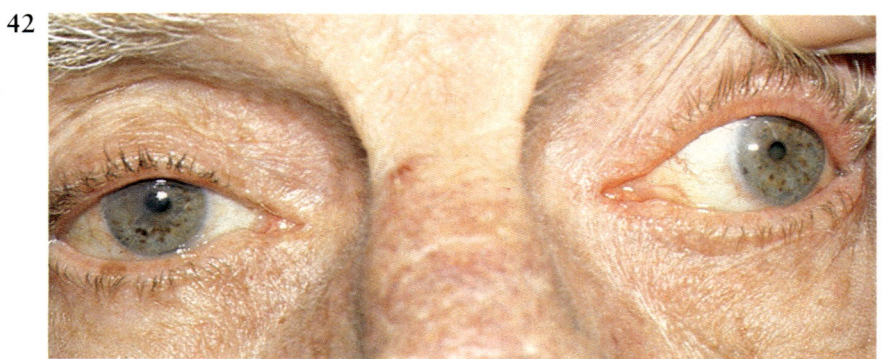

42 Partial left IIIrd nerve palsy with sparing of pupil.

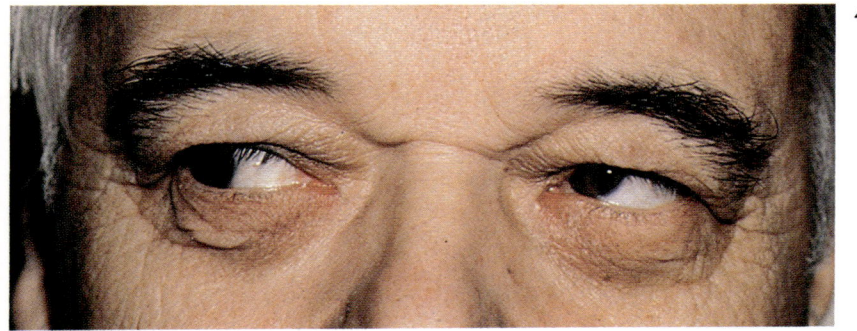

43 Left IVth nerve palsy. The left eye is higher than the right eye on adduction.

44 Bielschowsky head tilt test. This confirms a left IVth nerve palsy. When the head is tilted to the side of the palsy the eye on that side elevates as shown because of overaction of the superior rectus, now the principal intorter.

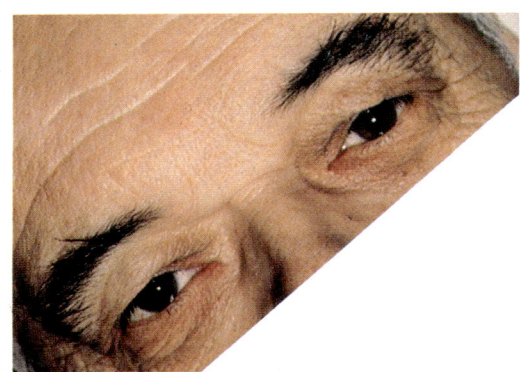

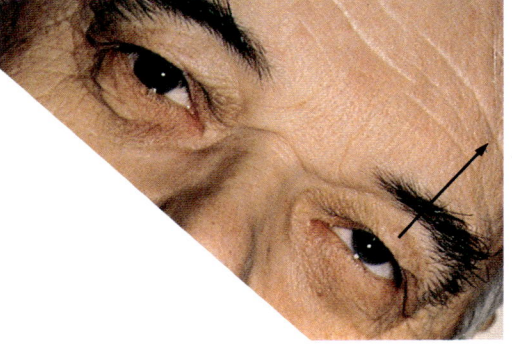

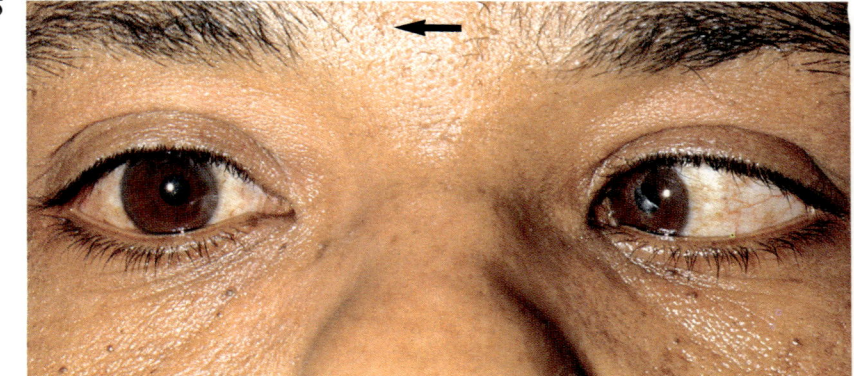

45 Right VIth nerve palsy.

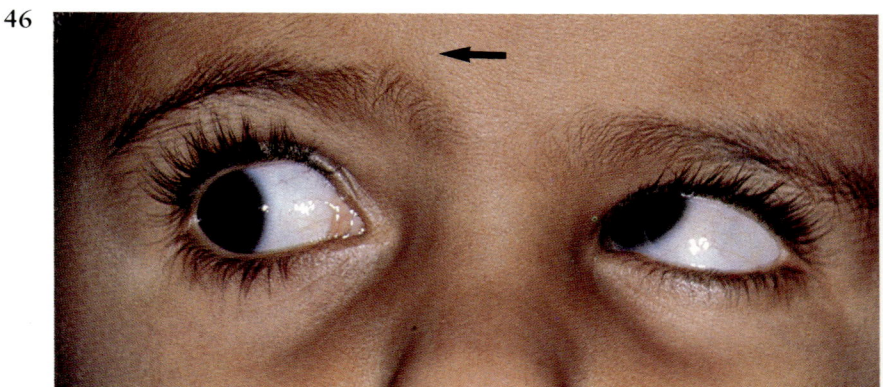

46 Left inferior oblique overaction. There is upshoot on adduction of the eye in which the overaction occurs.

The alternate cover test (Chapter 5) is helpful in the extremes of gaze to observe the relative deviation of the squinting and non-squinting eye and to discover in which direction of gaze the deviation is greatest.

Lid and pupil changes should also be observed, e.g. in Duane's syndrome there is narrowing of the palpebral fissure on adduction; in congenital or post-traumatic IIIrd nerve palsies with partial regeneration there may be pupil constriction on attempted adduction.

In the presence of a complete IIIrd nerve palsy, the eye will intort on attempted depression if the IVth nerve is still intact.

Where the defect does not fit a clear-cut pattern, diffuse muscle involvement such as occurs in thyrotoxicosis or orbital granuloma ('pseudotumour') should be considered.

In cases of non-paralytic strabismus, ductions (in which the movements of each eye are examined separately by covering the other eye) are initially full though the visual axes are not aligned. Later secondary changes may limit movement, e.g. a convergent eye may fail to abduct fully.

Supranuclear disorders

Pursuit movements are following movements and saccades are rapid eye movements. In addition to versions, pursuit and saccades are examined. Optokinetic nystagmus, the oculocephalic reflex and caloric responses are also elicited to study supranuclear control mechnisms but are not described here.

Pursuit
The eyes track a target moved slowly and uniformly a metre or more away from them. Abnormal pursuit velocity is detected by the presence of corrective saccades.

Saccades
The eyes move rapidly from one stationary target to another.

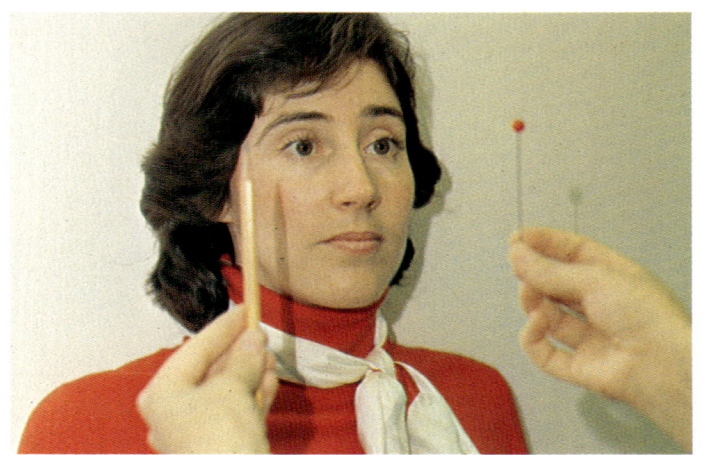

47 Saccades. Two differing targets are held before the patient e.g. a red pin immediately in front and a pencil to the right, 30° to 40° apart. The patient is asked to fix the pin initially.

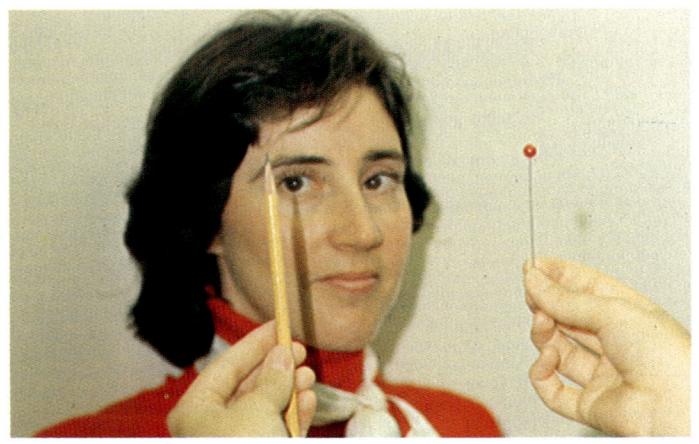

48 Saccades. On the command 'pencil' the patient looks at the pencil. During the lateral version the examiner watches the eye movements. This is repeated several times (i.e. 'pin', 'pencil', 'pin', etc.) to permit exact observation. It is then repeated for the other side with the second target (e.g. pencil) to the left.

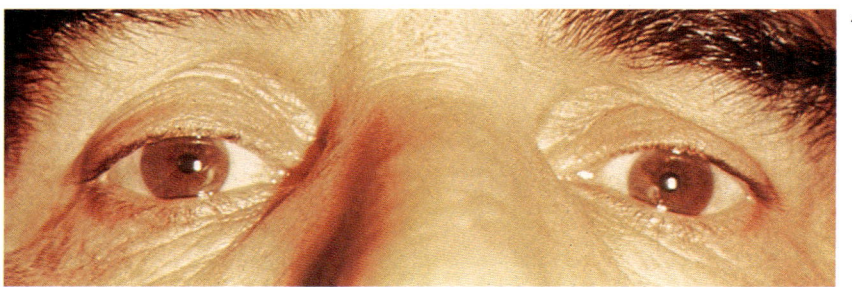

49 Right internuclear ophthalmoplegia (primary position). The adduction defect in an internuclear ophthalmoplegia is best illustrated by examining saccadic movements, though it is also present to pursuit. Convergence may be normal.

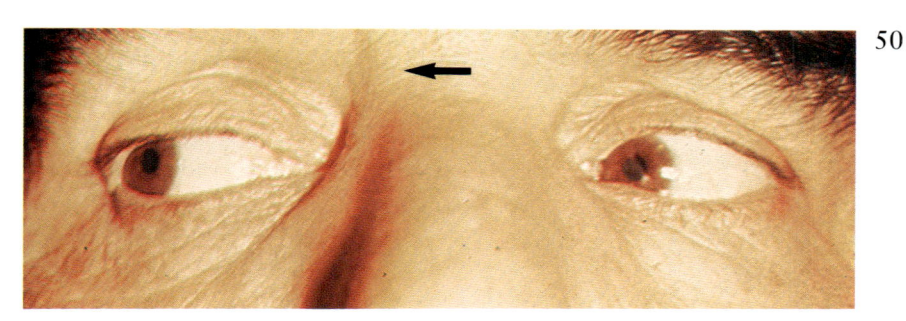

50 Right internuclear ophthalmoplegia (dextroversion). Normal right abduction and left adduction.

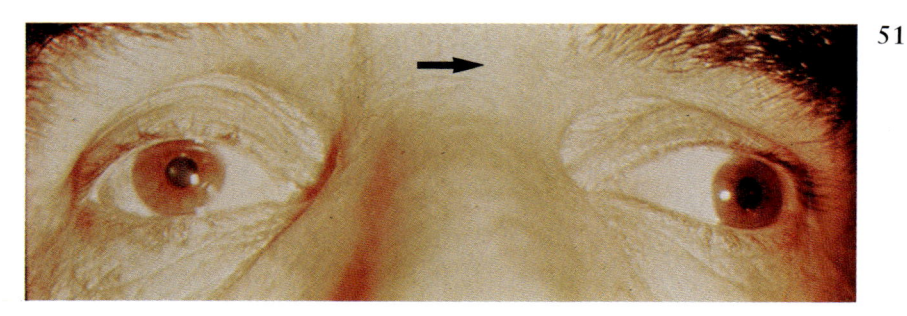

51 Right internuclear ophthalmoplegia (levoversion). The right eye fails to adduct. There is nystagmus of the abducting left eye.

Lid measurements

Ptosis
Quantative assessment is necessary to monitor the progress of disease over time. Both sides should be measured even if only one side appears affected.

52 Measurement of ptosis. The patient's head is positioned normally. If wrinkling of the forehead suggests frontalis action, it is prevented by firm backward and downward pressure on the brow. The patient looks straight ahead and the vertical height of the palpebral fissure is measured in front of the pupil.

This method depends on the lower lid and globe being in a normal position and the examiner must consider lower lid abnormalities or enophthalmos as sources of inaccuracy. The distance between the upper lid margin and the corneal reflex or limbus also provides a measure of ptosis and the technique used should be indicated with a diagram. A photograph provides a permanent record.

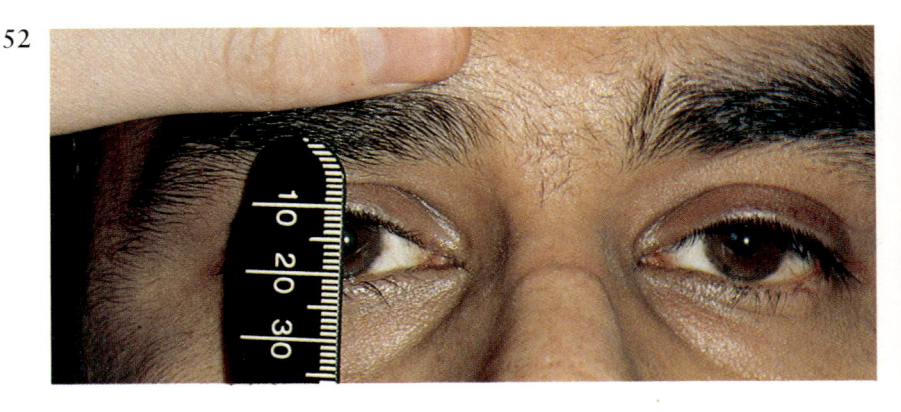

Levator function (relevant to ptosis surgery)

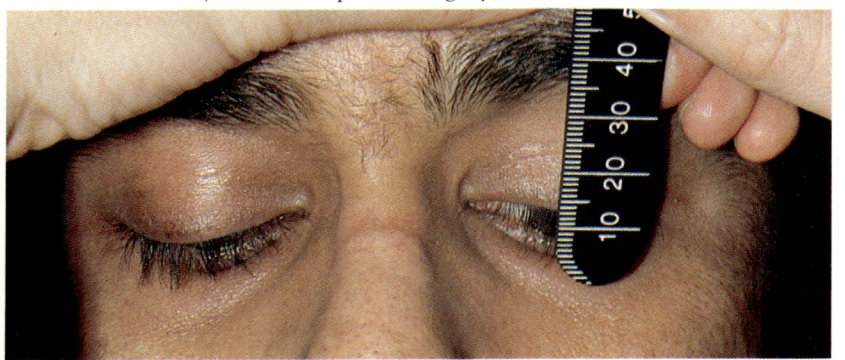

53 Levator function. The patient's head is positioned normally and frontalis overaction is prevented by firm pressure over the brow. A ruler is held before the upper lid in full downgaze and the marking on the ruler at the upper lid margin is noted.

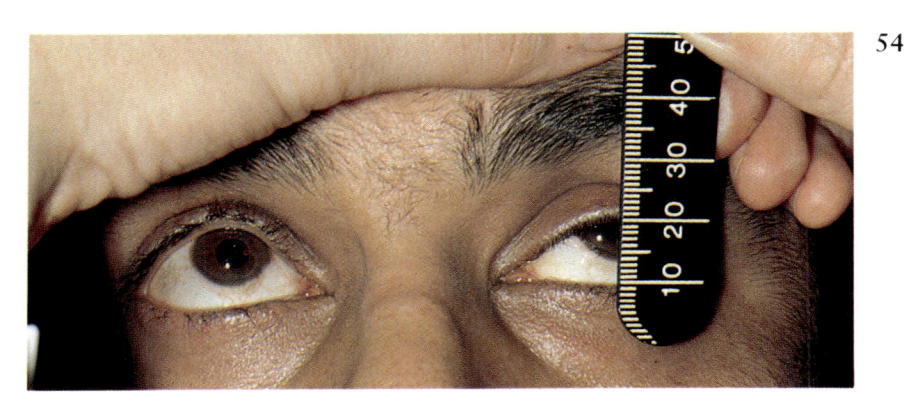

54 Levator function. The patient then gazes fully up (without moving his head) and the excursion of the lid in millimetres seen on the ruler is recorded. (Normal 15-18 mm.)

Corneal reflex

Corneal anaesthesia is relevant to both neuro-ophthalmology (Vth nerve) and corneal disease.

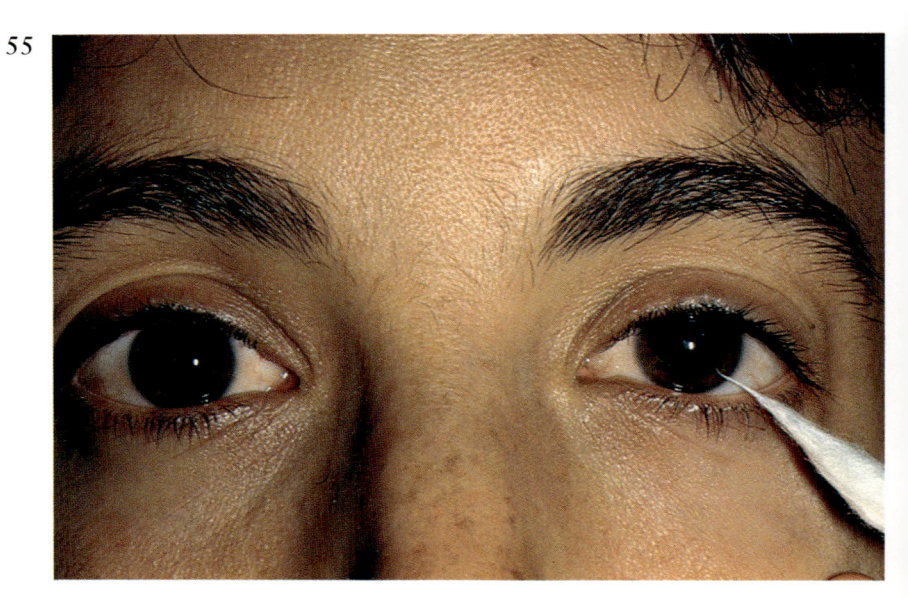

55 Corneal reflex. A piece of clean cotton wool drawn into a thread-like point is used (firmer materials may abrade the cornea). The eye is approached from the side to avoid a startle reflex. The lids and lashes should also be avoided. The cornea is lightly touched outside the visual axis and may result in a blink, or the examiner can ask the patient if he feels the sensation. This is compared to the other eye, touching the corresponding point on the cornea. The sensitivity of the normal cornea decreases going away from the centre. There are formal aesthesiometers available with a filament tip and a gauge, e.g. the Cochet and Bonnet instrument.

Orbital examination

Measurement of the degree of proptosis (forward movement of the globe in relation to the bony orbit), and horizontal and vertical displacement of the globe, are appropriate where orbital pathology is suspected.

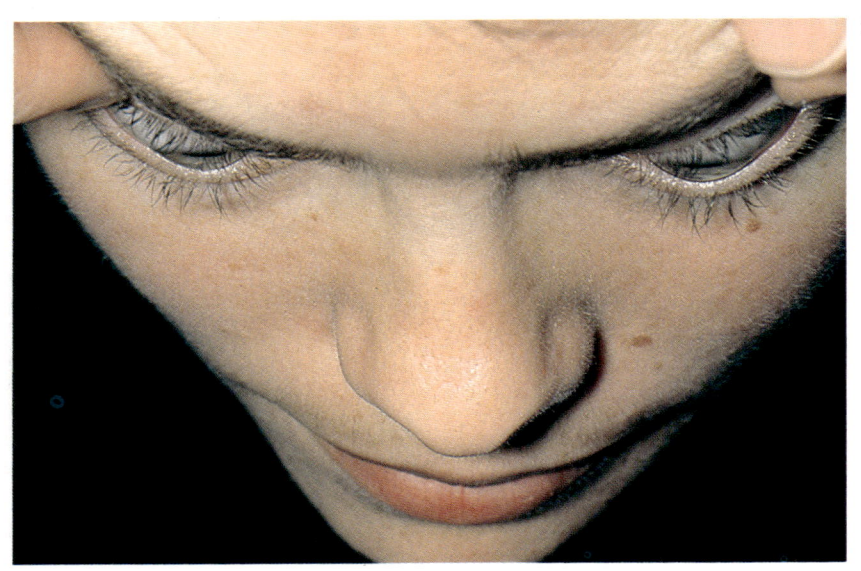

56 Qualitative examination. Proptosis may be observed by standing behind the seated patient, raising the upper lids, and comparing the protrusion of each globe when the patient looks downwards. A more quantitative method is provided by exophthalmometry.

Exophthalmometry

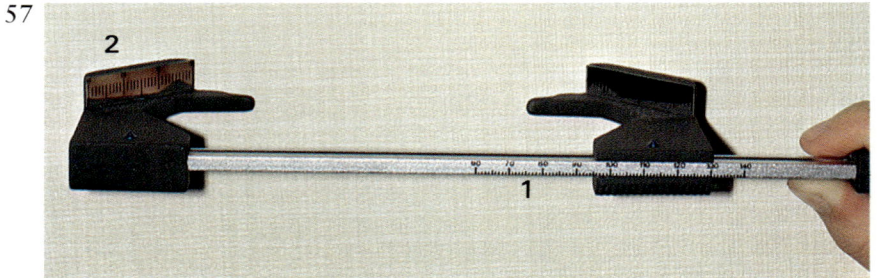

57 Hertel-type exophthalmometer. The instrument has a scale to measure the distance between the lateral canthi (1) and a scale on either side to measure the protrusion of each eye (2).

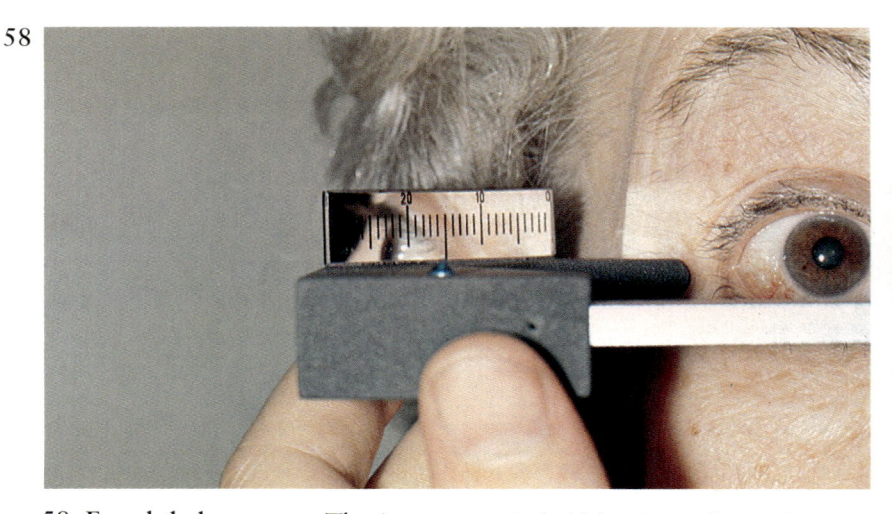

58 Exophthalmometry. The instrument is held horizontally in front of the eyes with the 45° mirrors upwards. The intercanthal distance is adjusted so that the instrument rests on both lateral orbital rims at the level of the outer canthi. The appropriate vertical markers, here a blue stud and a long vertical line in the centre of the proptosis scale, are aligned, and the reading from the lateral orbital rim to the corneal apex is taken—it is 24 mm here. This is repeated for the other eye.

The results are recorded as follows:

```
        (Intercanthal distance)
              109
     ┌─────────────────┐
    24                20
  (right)           (left)
```

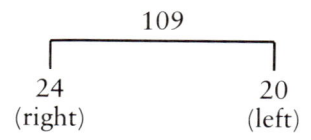

A difference of more than 2 mm between the eyes is thought to be significant. The distance between the lateral canthi must be recorded to permit consistent future readings to be taken at the same separation.

The degree of exophthalmos may be objectively recorded with a lateral photograph of the eye showing a reference rule held horizontally from the lateral orbital rim.

Displacement from axis

Masses outside the muscle cone may displace the eye vertically or horizontally, e.g. a frontal sinus mucocele will displace the eye down and outwards. Masses within the muscle cone tend to cause an axial proptosis without vertical or horizontal displacement.

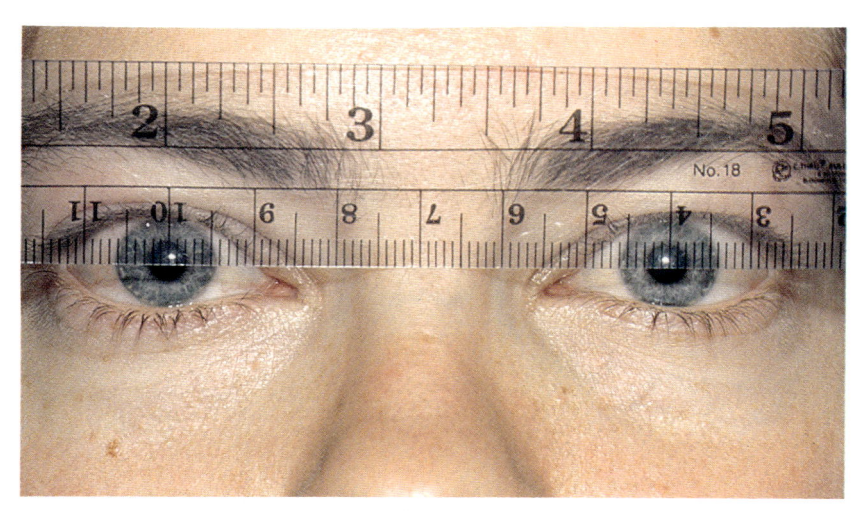

59 Displacement. The patient's eyes are in the primary position. The ruler is placed horizontally along the outer canthi.

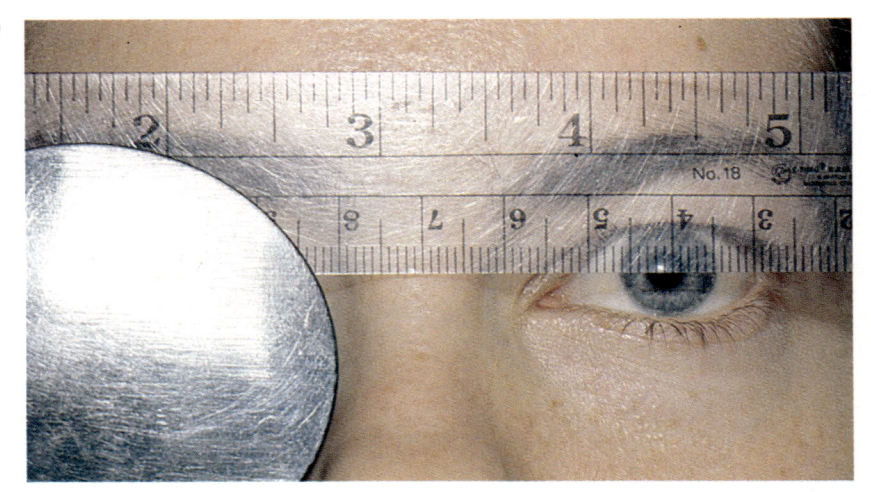

60 Displacement. The other eye is occluded or a squint may produce erroneous results. Differences in the vertical distance from the ruler to the lower limbus indicates vertical displacement. Horizontal displacement is measured from the presumed midline of the face, i.e. the middle of the bridge of the nose, to the nasal limbus. This is recorded with a diagram.

To distinguish between neurogenic and mechanical causes of eye movement abnormality in orbital pathology, the intra-ocular pressure can be measured with the eye looking away from the involved muscle and compared to the pressure in the primary position. An increase suggests compression of the globe by a tethered muscle. In the forced duction test, the anaesthetized eye is passively moved with forceps, and restriction of movement is confirmed.

Radiology

X-rays and CT (computerized tomography) scans are indispensable to neuro-ophthalmology. More recently MRI (magnetic resonance imaging) scans have also become available. The new generation scans provide such high resolution that tomograms and angiograms are less frequently required for diagnosis.

X-rays

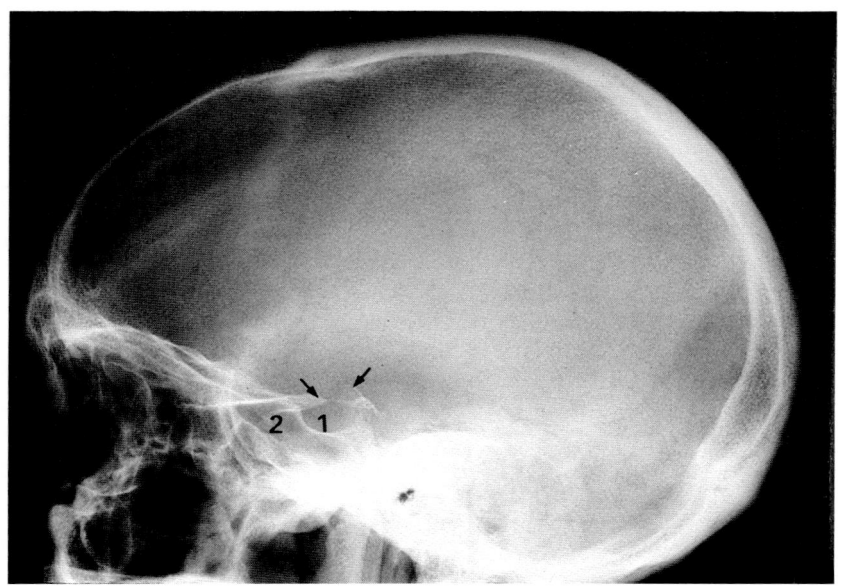

61 Lateral skull X-ray, normal. Note the pituitary fossa (1), the anterior and posterior clinoid processes (arrows), and the sphenoid sinus (2).

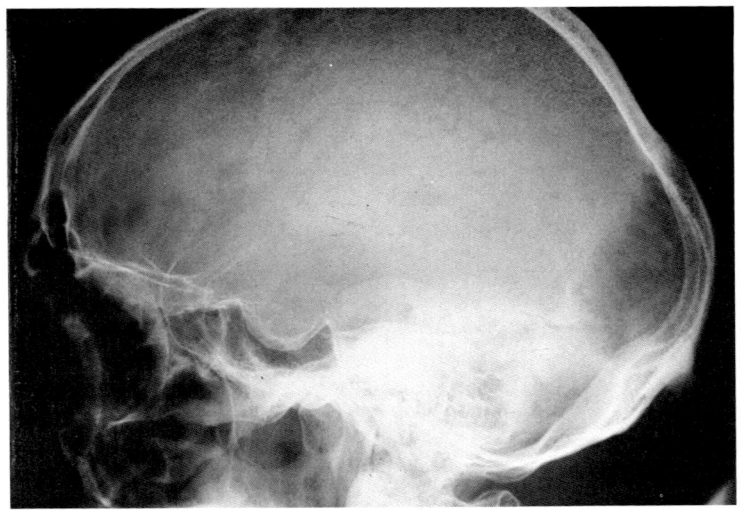

62 Lateral skull X-ray, pituitary tumour. The pituitary fossa is grossly enlarged and the clinoid processes are eroded.

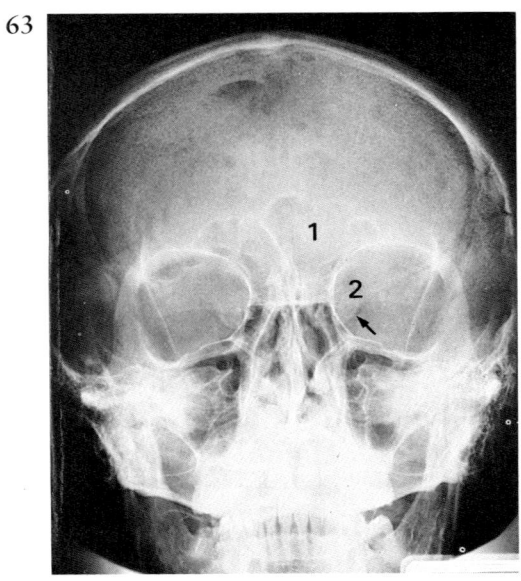

63 PA skull X-ray. Note the normal frontal sinus (1), sphenoid ridge (2), and the superior orbital fissure (arrow).

64 Orbital views. A normal optic foramen is clearly shown (arrow). Other orbital views illustrate different features, but high resolution CT scanning is superseding these.

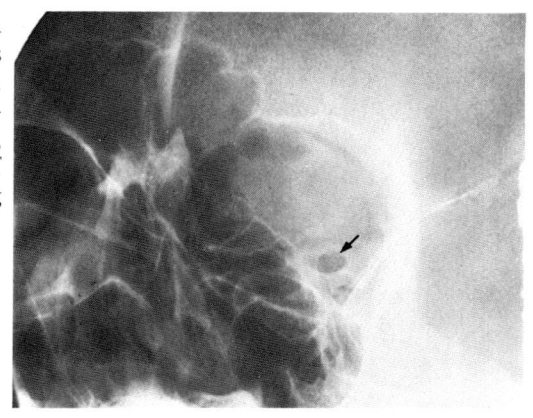

CT scans

CT scans should be both unenhanced and enhanced, i.e. both without and with the injection of intravenous contrast medium (unless contraindications exist), otherwise an isodense space occupying lesion cannot be excluded. Both head and orbital scans may be performed.

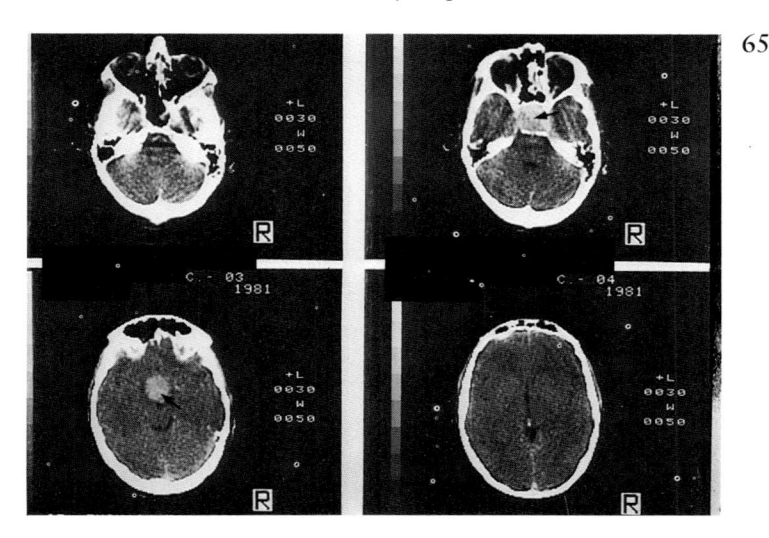

65 CT scan of head (1981)—enhanced. Axial sections at level of pituitary fossa. A pituitary tumour is apparent (arrows).

45

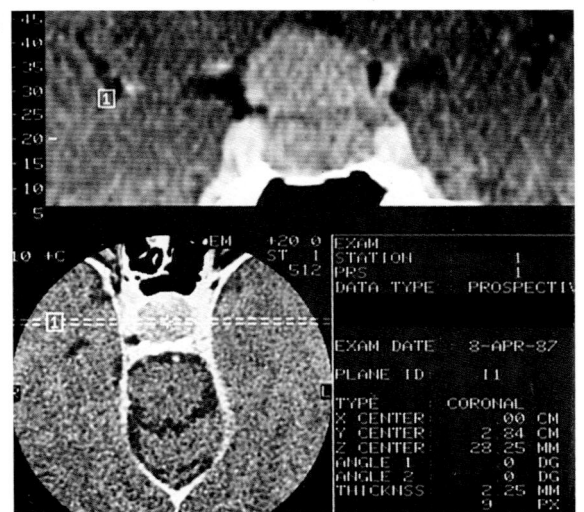

66 CT scan of head (1987)—enhanced. The axial scan shows a pituitary tumour. The data is reconstructed by the computer into the coronal section shown above the axial scan. The tumour is seen rising above the sella.

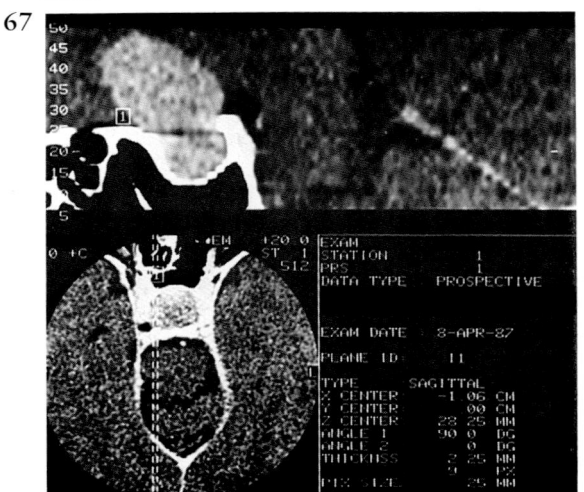

67 CT scan of head—enhanced. Sagittal reconstruction in the same case as 66.

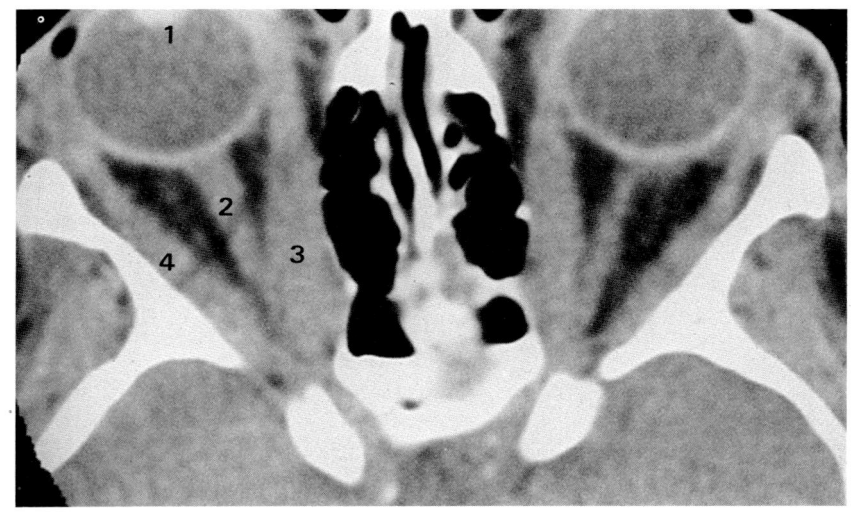

68 CT scan of orbit—enhanced. Dysthyroid eye disease. Note the lens (1), the optic nerve (2), the thickened medial rectus (3) and lateral rectus (4).

MRI scans

Magnetic resonance imaging is a method of visualizing intracranial structures without ionizing radiation or intravenous injections. As yet its availability is limited. Patients with metal prostheses or cardiac pacemakers are excluded. CT scanning is still the preferred method of imaging the orbit.

69 MRI scan—sagittal section. Mild enlargement of the pituitary (arrow). Bone yields a low signal and so seems invisible, whereas fat yields a high signal intensity and appears bright.

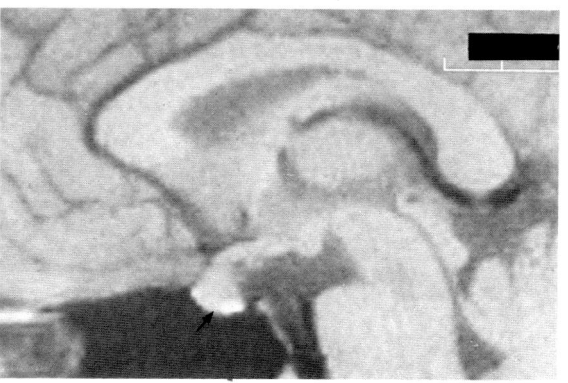

Electrodiagnosis

Accepted methods for recording the electro-oculogram (EOG), electroretinogram (ERG), or visual evoked potential (VEP) vary. There is an extensive literature describing a variety of stimuli, recording conditions, recording methods and interpretation of ocular electrodiagnosis. Only basic examples are considered here.

Electro-oculogram
The eye forms an electrical dipole with a potential difference of several millivolts, sustained by the retinal pigment epithelium, between the cornea (positive) and the back of the eye (negative). Normally this potential at least doubles from the dark-adapted to the light-adapted state (the light rise). Static electrodes placed, for example, at the canthi, measure the change in potential presented to them by voluntary horizontal gaze excursions of the ocular dipole.

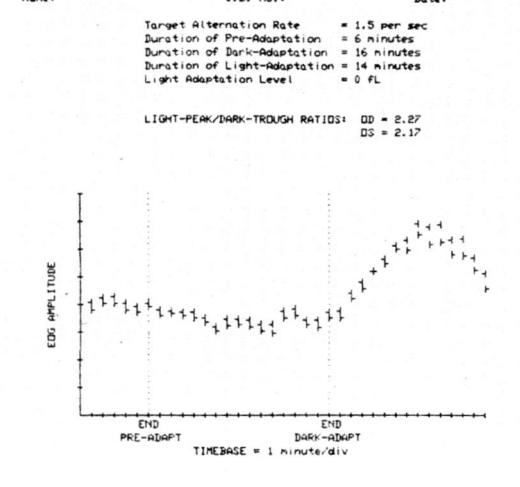

70 EOG, normal tracing. The right eye is indicated by a vertical line with a crossbar to the right, the left with the crossbar to the left.

ELECTRO-OCULOGRAM

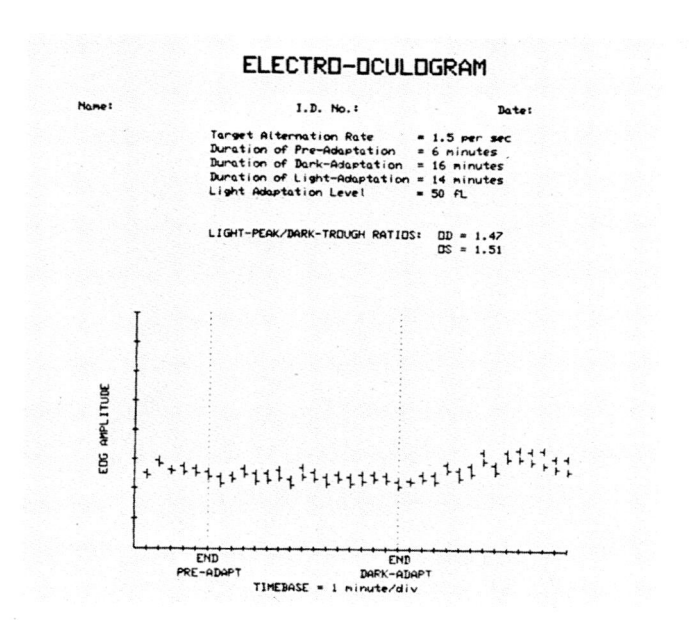

Name: I.D. No.:   Date:

Target Alternation Rate   = 1.5 per sec
Duration of Pre-Adaptation   = 6 minutes
Duration of Dark-Adaptation   = 16 minutes
Duration of Light-Adaptation   = 14 minutes
Light Adaptation Level   = 50 fL

LIGHT-PEAK/DARK-TROUGH RATIOS: OD = 1.47
                                 OS = 1.51

TIMEBASE = 1 minute/div

71 EOG. Tracing in a patient with Best's vitelliform macular dystrophy in which the normal light rise is absent.

Electroretinogram

Stimulation of the retina with light results in an action potential superimposed on the resting potential which can be measured by a corneal electrode (frequently gold foil) and an indifferent electrode, e.g. on the forehead. A single flash stimulus is followed after a latent period by a negative deflection (a-wave) and a positive deflection (b-wave) superimposed on which may be oscillations (oscillatory potentials). The entire response is usually less than 250 milliseconds. The flash ERG is a mass response of the outer layers of the retina and is subnormal when the retina is extensively diseased. The use of a pattern stimulus is still largely restricted to research.

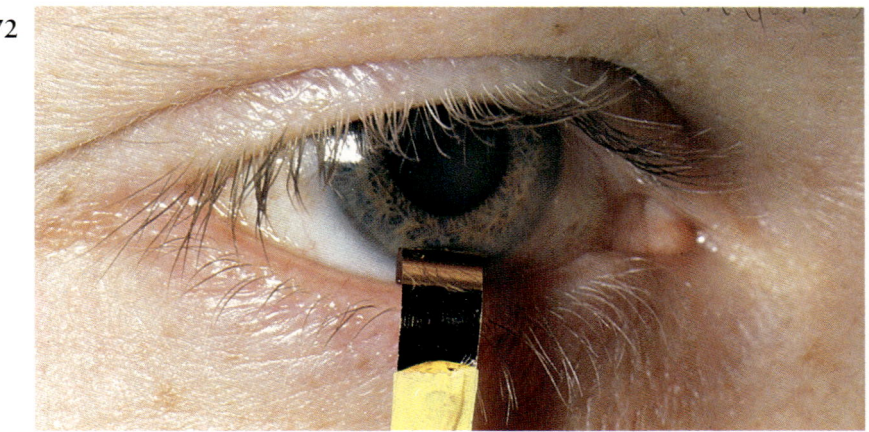

72 ERG. A gold foil corneal electrode.

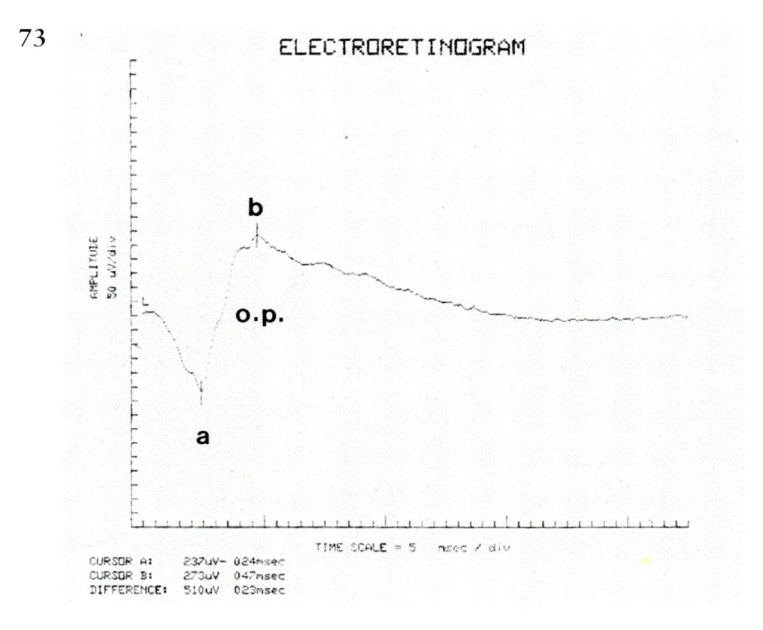

73 Flash ERG, normal. The a-wave, b-wave and oscillatory potentials are seen.

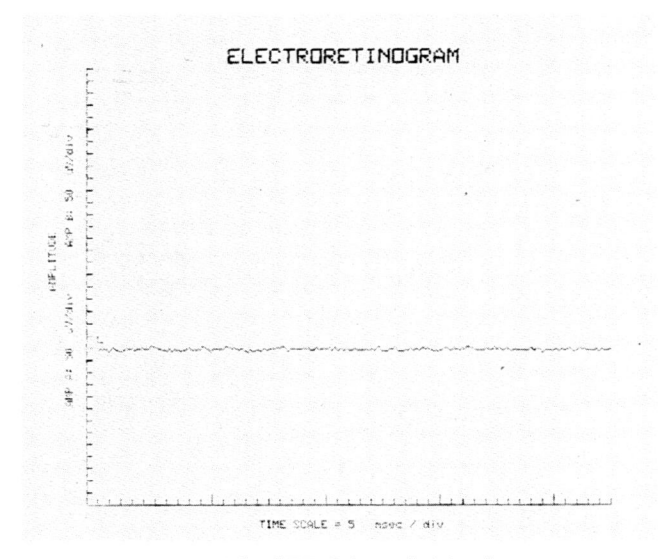

74 ERG. Extinguished ERG in retinitis pigmentosa.

Visual evoked potential (response)
Multiple flash or checkerboard pattern stimuli are presented to the subject as the occipital pole electro-encephalogram is recorded. Computer averaging cancels out other cerebral activity allowing definition of the visual evoked potential. A positive deflection occurs about 120 msec after a pattern stimulus.

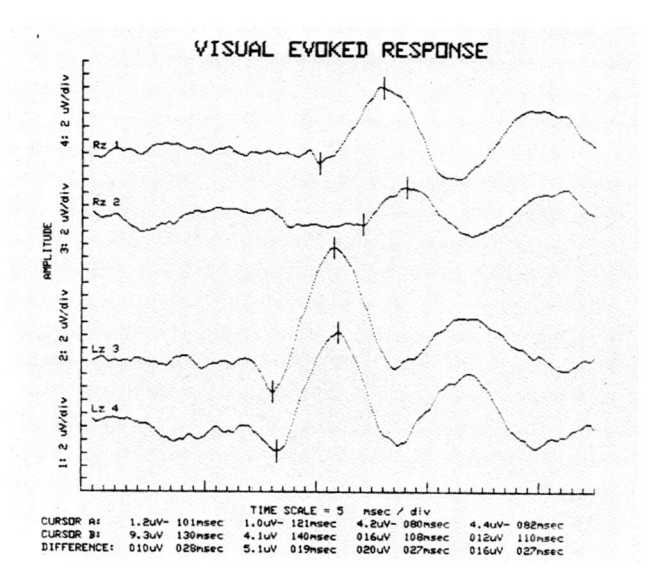

75 VEP—pattern stimulus. Two tracings are shown from each eye. The lower tracings show a response of normal latency and amplitude (for the laboratory concerned). The upper tracings show an increased latency and decreased amplitude of the main peak due to retrobulbar neuritis. The latency will remain increased even if vision and visual fields return to normal.

5 Tests for squint

The cover-uncover test is used to diagnose a manifest squint (tropia) and to determine the fixing eye. If no tropia is found, the alternate cover test is performed and a latent squint (phoria) may be elicited.

Cover-uncover test

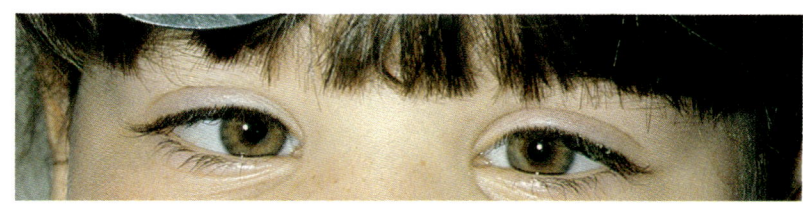

76 Cover-uncover test. The primary position. The patient is asked to fix a distant target or a light (which provides a non-accommodative target). The eye which is to remain uncovered is observed.

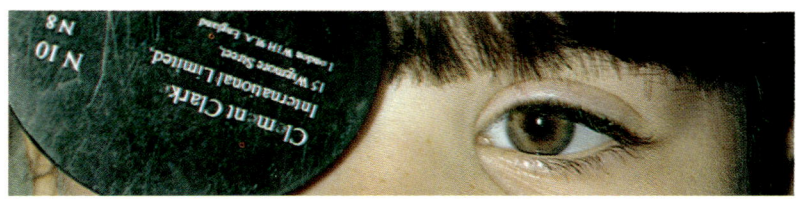

77 Cover-uncover test. The right eye is covered. The left eye does not move. The left eye is therefore fixing on the distant target as it does not move to take up fixation.

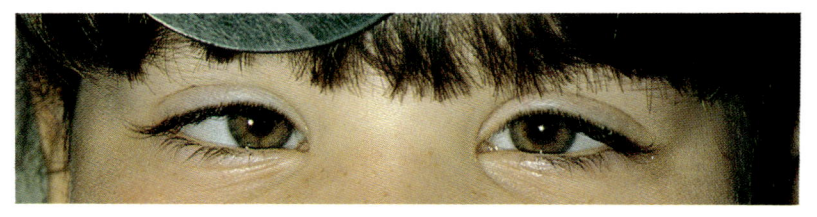

78 Cover-uncover test. The cover is removed, permitting attempted binocular vision again.

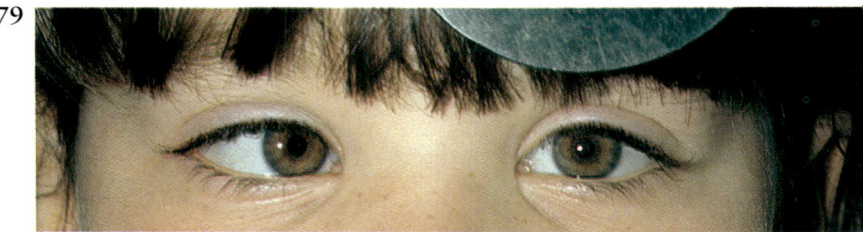

79 Cover-uncover test. The cover crosses the forehead to the other side.

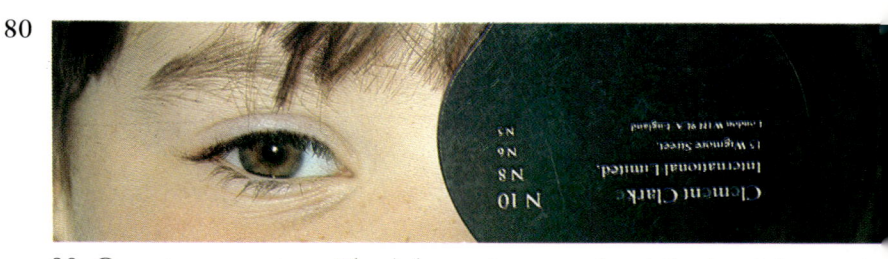

80 Cover-uncover test. The left eye is covered, while the right eye is observed. The right eye is seen to move to take up fixation. It was therefore not fixing before, during attempted binocular gaze. Thus a manifest squint exists, in this case a right convergent squint. On removing the cover altogether, the left eye takes up fixation again and the right eye returns to its convergent position as in 76.

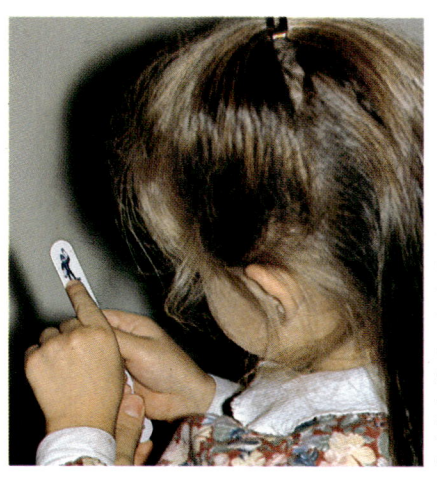

81 Accommodative squint. Children are asked about small details on an accommodative target, e.g. 'How many buttons on the policeman's coat?', to elicit an accommodative component in a squint. A cover-uncover test is performed and repeated with a full hypermetropic correction to determine improvement.

Alternate cover test

In this test the occluder is swung from one eye to the other so that both eyes cannot fix simultaneously and so their positions are not determined by the need for fusion.

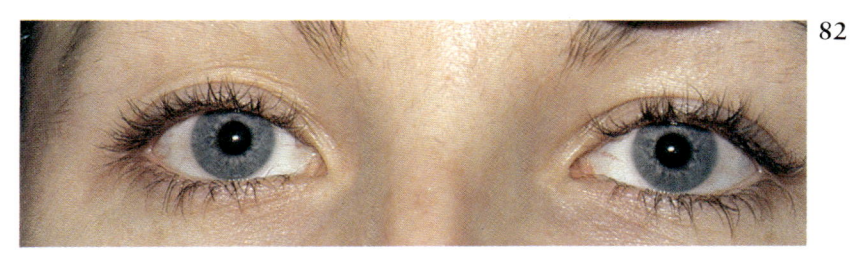

82 Alternate cover test. The eyes are straight in the primary position. A distant target or a light is fixed.

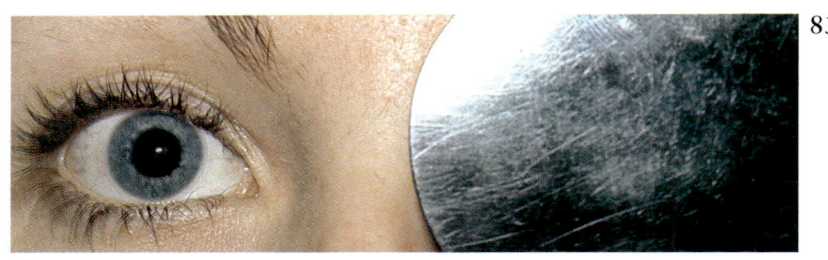

83 Alternate cover test. One eye is occluded, e.g. the left. The eye being occluded is watched (unlike the cover-uncover test).

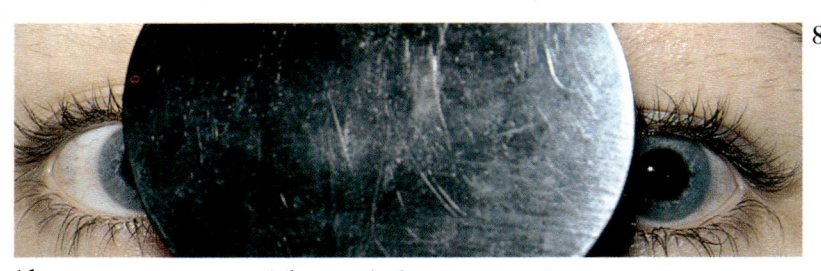

84 Alternate cover test. The occluder is moved across the nose to occlude the right eye. The eyes are thus dissociated. The left eye has diverged behind the occluder in the absence of the stimulus to fusion (the corneal reflex is no longer central).

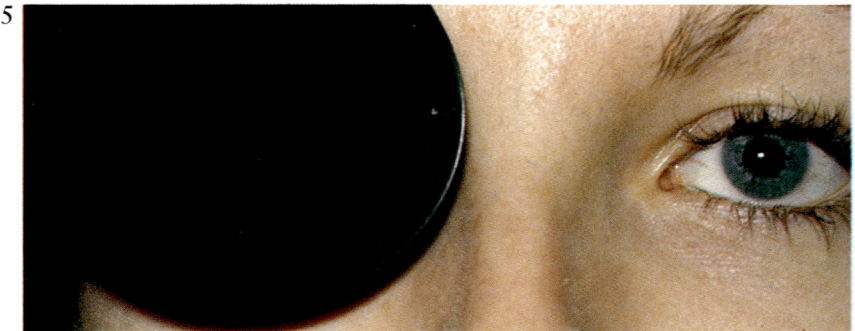

85 Alternate cover test. The left eye takes up fixation.

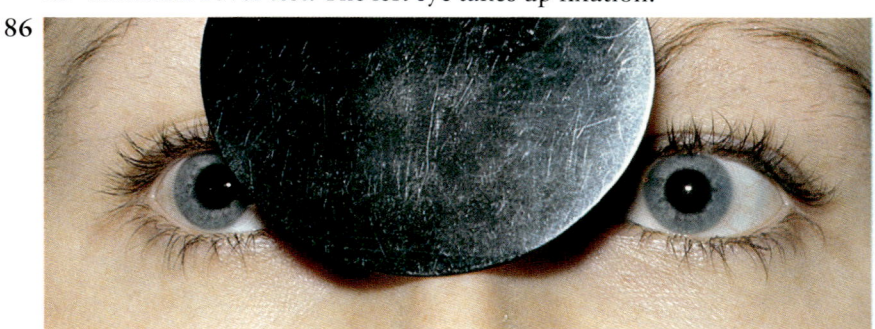

86 Alternate cover test. The occluder is moved back to the left and the right eye is seen to have diverged under the occluder.

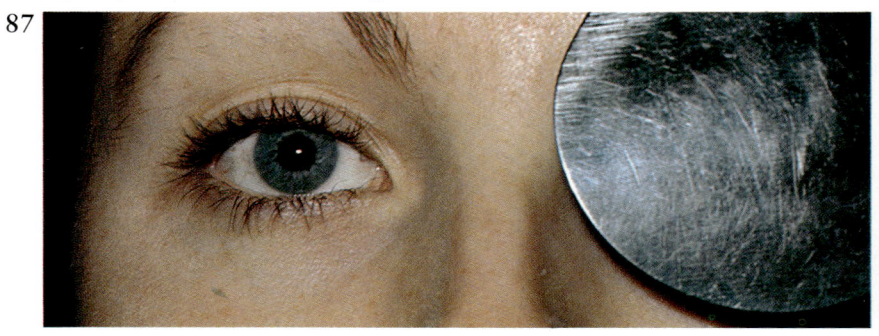

87 Alternate cover test. The right eye takes up fixation. This is a latent divergent squint.

Prism cover test

This is the alternate cover test performed with a prism over one eye with the aim of reducing the movement of the eye taking up fixation to a minimum. The angle of squint can thus be quantified.

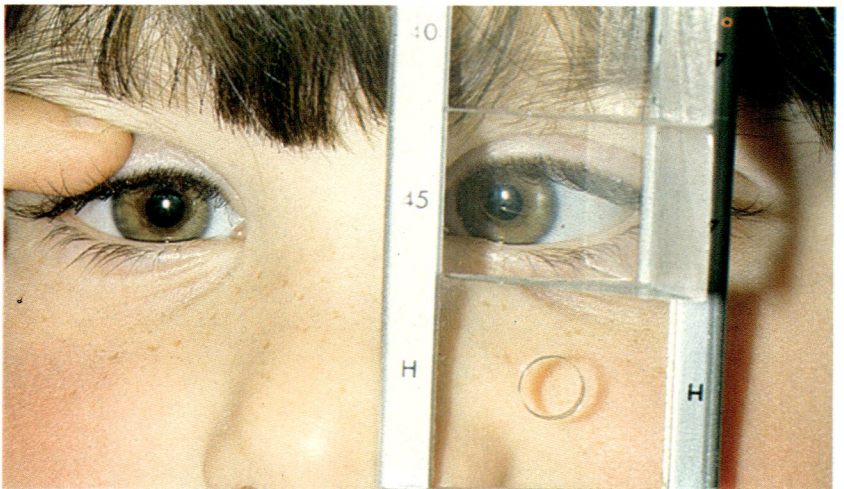

88 Prism cover test. Prisms of increasing strength are placed before one eye, with the apex in the direction of deviation, and the alternate cover test is performed until movements to take up fixation no longer occur, i.e. the images reaching the two eyes are aligned. The corneal reflex can be observed as a guide to the end-point in patients with amblyopia or poor fixation, and in infants. When it falls on the same part of the pupil as in the fixing eye, alignment has been attained.

Both manifest and latent components of the squint are included in this result. It is performed for distance, and near, using an accommodative target. An assistant may be needed to handle prism, occluder and target.

The advantage of the prism cover test over the major amblyoscope is that it is performed in dynamic circumstances with continued dissociation of the eyes. It is the best way to measure intermittent squints and is the measurement on which surgery is usually based. The method is less suitable for combined horizontal and vertical deviations and cannot measure torsion.

Fixation

This may be central or eccentric. The cover-uncover test demonstrates which eye is squinting. The nature of fixation in that eye can be determined using a direct ophthalmoscope with a fixation graticule that may be seen projected onto the retina. The eye not being examined must be occluded. The examiner looks at the fundus through the ophthalmoscope and the patient is asked to look at the target. Pupillary dilatation may be required. If the shadow of the fixation device falls on the fovea, fixation is central; if it falls elsewhere, fixation is eccentric. The patient may not immediately find the fixation point due to reduced acuity. (NB. The light intensity must be low for the fixation device to be seen by the patient.)

Four dioptre prism test

This is useful in microtropias, i.e. squints of 8 prism dioptres or less with a suppression scotoma and a form of binocular vision, but there is a proportion of patients that respond negatively to this test.

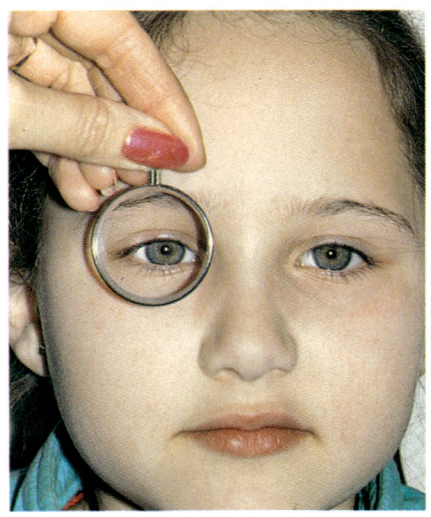

89 Four dioptre prism test. If a 4 dioptre prism is placed base out (apex in) before an eye that is fixing, that eye will adduct to restore fixation. If the other eye has normal fixation it will abduct briefly, as the contralateral synergist acts, then adduct again to restore alignment. Abnormal responses are : (1) no movement at all, i.e. the image has fallen on a suppression scotoma in the eye behind the prism; or (2) a single abduction movement of the other eye but no realignment, i.e. a scotoma in the other eye prevents diplopia occurring.

Binocular vision

90 Infants. When an 8 dioptre base out prism is placed in front of one eye of an infant of six months or over, convergence will result if single binocular vision is present. (A central corneal reflex indicates fixation.)

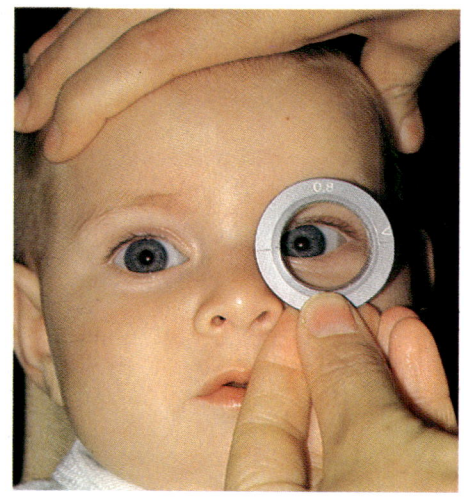

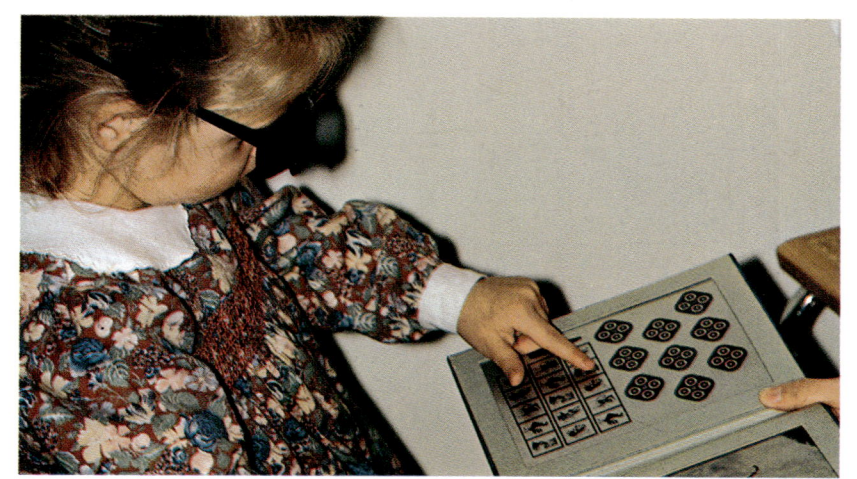

91 Stereograms—Titmus test. A child with good single binocular vision wearing the test glasses will be able to identify or reach for the three-dimensional object perceived in the stereo illustrations. Grades of stereopsis can be determined with various sets of stereograms.

Major amblyoscope

The major amblyoscope (synoptophore) consists of two tubes mounted so that they can be moved in any plane, with an illuminated slot at the end of each tube where a variety of targets can be inserted. Each eye looks down a separate tube, the optics of which do not require accommodation for the targets to be seen clearly. The examiner aligns the corneal reflexes in the pupils and is then able to read the angle of deviation on a scale. He can perform a cover test by alternately illuminating each target and asking the patient to look from one to the other, adjusting the angle of the tubes until there is no movement of the eyes. Horizontal inaccuracies may occur due to unnecessary accommodation and its associated convergence. Vertical and torsional deviations are accurately measured.

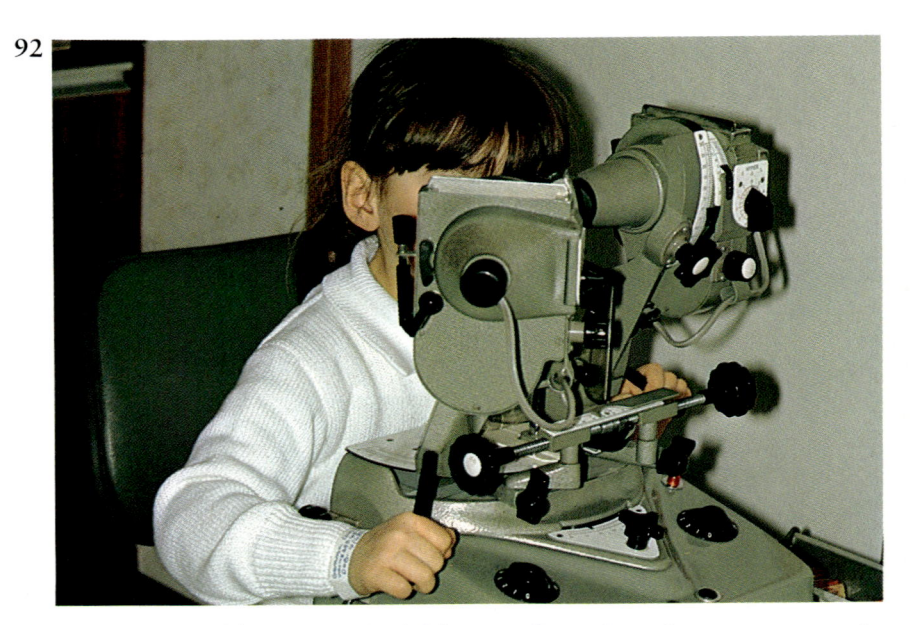

92 Major amblyoscope. A child can adjust the tubes to arrange the pictures appropriately, e.g. putting a goldfish seen by one eye into a bowl seen by the other eye. The major amblyoscope can be used to study degrees of fusion by using appropriate combinations of targets.

Hess charts

These are useful in investigating ocular muscle imbalance, both paretic and non-paretic. The eyes are dissociated either by red-green goggles or by a mirror, and the patient is asked to put a marker, visible only with one eye on a dot visible only with the other. For example, if he has a right sixth nerve palsy, while fixing on the dot in the right temporal field with his right eye, his left medial rectus will overact due to conjugate innervation. He will therefore place the marker seen with the left eye too far over to the right, past the dot which is invisible to his left eye. The points where the marker is placed are recorded and the procedure is repeated fixing with the left eye. The smaller field belongs to the eye with the paresis and in this field, maximum displacement from the normal cardinal position in the chart is produced by the palsied muscle.

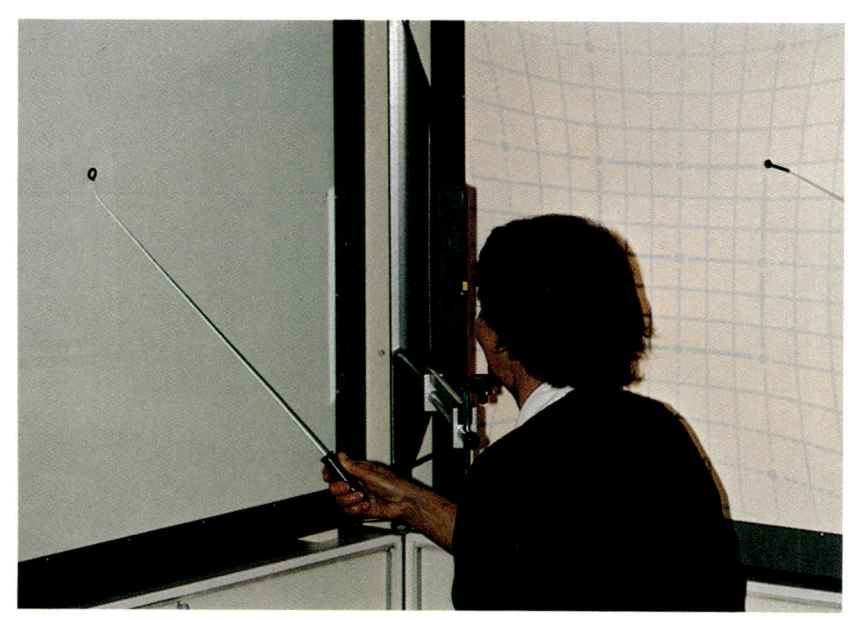

93 Charting muscle imbalance. The patient's eyes are dissociated by a mirror. The right eye looks at the chart straight ahead and the left eye views a mirror image of the chart on the left.

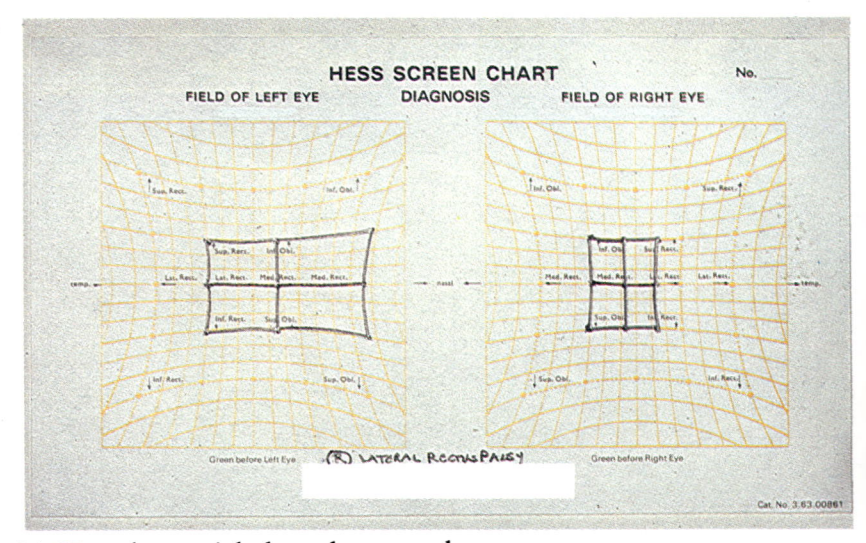

94 Hess chart—right lateral rectus palsy.

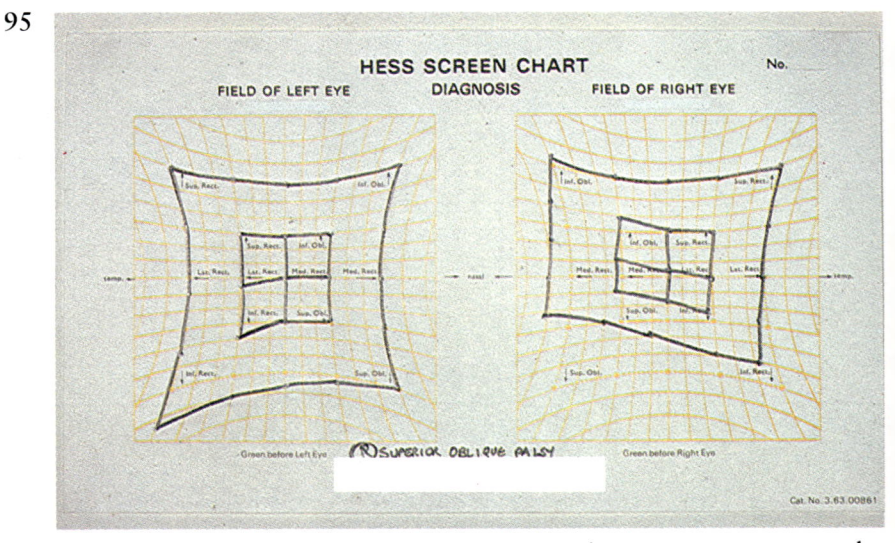

95 Hess chart—right superior oblique palsy. The outer square may only be plotted if the defect is subtle.

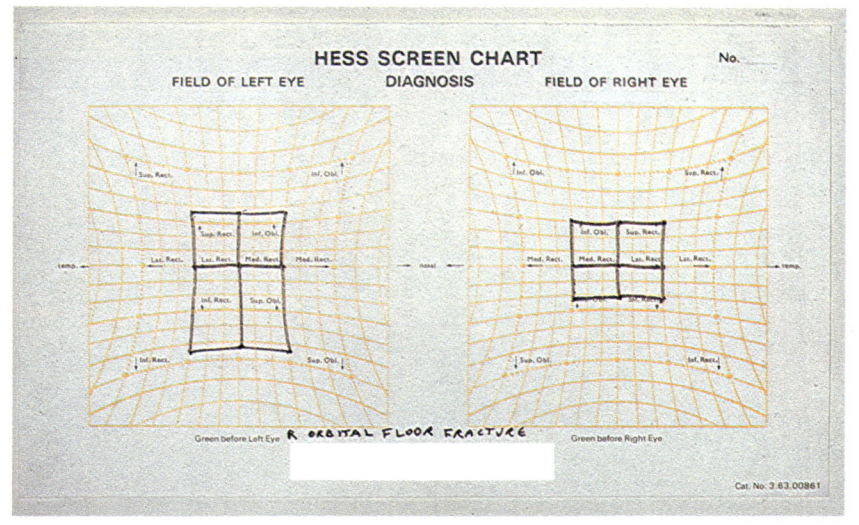

96 Hess chart—blowout fracture of right orbit (mechanical restriction).

6 Tests of lacrimal function

Tear production

The tear film breakup time (BUT) assesses the stability of the tear film and a decreased BUT implies that the tears are mucin deficient.

The principal test for aqueous production is the Schirmer test. This is used to determine the lacrimal secretion over five minutes and is most commonly required in diagnosis of dry eyes.

Tear film BUT
This is performed before the instillation of any drops, particularly local anaesthetic. The patient's lids must not be held open by the examiner. The inferior tarsal conjunctiva is touched with a moistened fluorescein strip, and the patient blinks several times to spread the dye, then looks straight ahead. The time from a complete blink to the appearance of the first randomly distributed defect (black spot), observed with the slit lamp using the blue filter and diffuse illumination, is the BUT. A BUT greater than or equal to 10 seconds is said to be normal.

Schirmer test
The standard Schirmer test (No. 1) is performed without local anaesthetic. (The Schirmer No. 2 test requires stimulation of the nasal mucosa and is not often performed.)

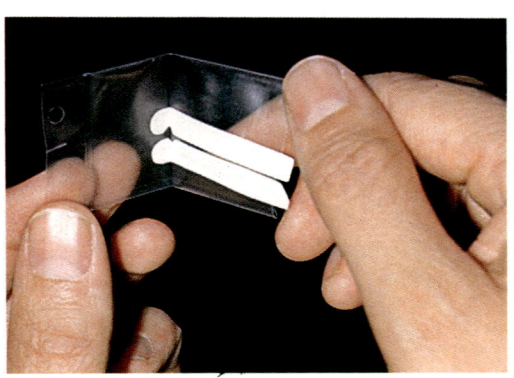

97 Schirmer test. The test strips are bent at right angles at the indentation within the plastic container to keep the strips clean.

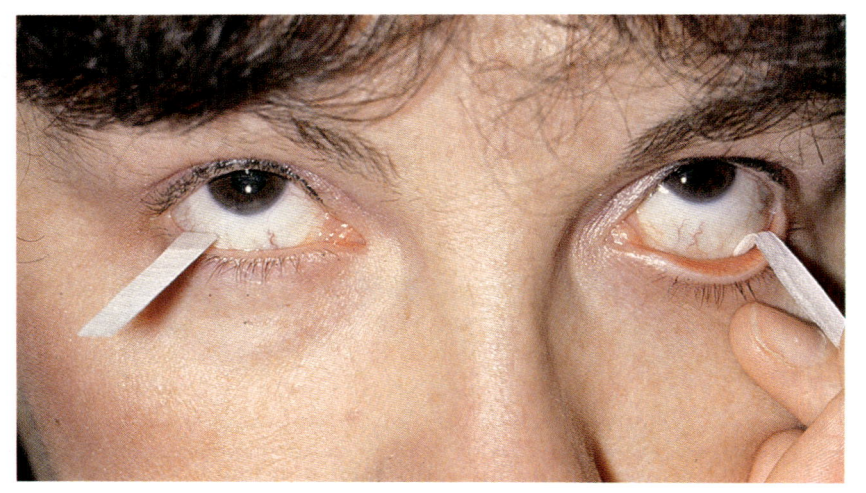

98 Schirmer test. The patient looks up, the lower lid is drawn down, and a test strip is inserted into the lower fornix laterally in both eyes. This must be done gently without touching the cornea. The patient can look ahead and continue to blink normally.

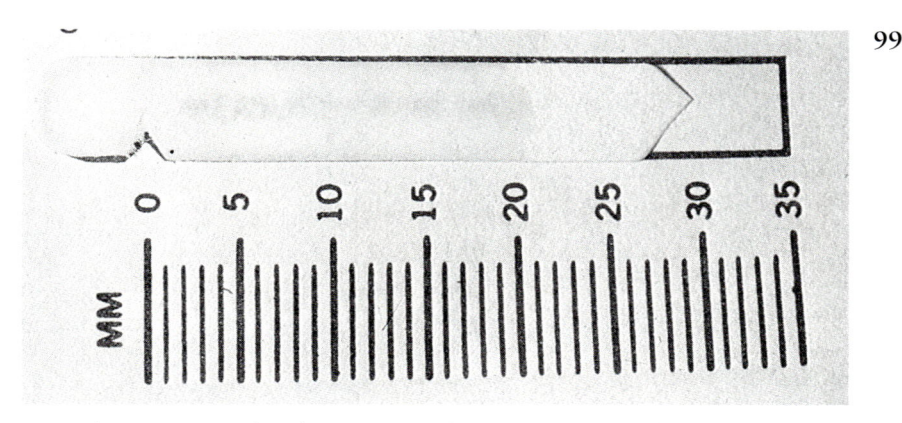

99 Schirmer test. After five minutes the strip is removed and the distance that the fluid has reached from the indentation is measured in millimetres. Over 15 mm of wetting measured from the indentation is normal and lower readings may be normal in the elderly. Less than 5 mm is always abnormal.

The basic secretion test of Jones
If the conjunctiva and cornea are anaesthetized prior to insertion of the filter paper, the basic secretion from the glands of Krause and Wolfring is measured rather than the reflex secretion from the lacrimal gland. Less than 8 mm of wetting measured from the indentation is abnormal.

Cotton thread measurement of basic secretion
Cotton thread impregnated with phenol red indicator and inserted into the inferior fornix for 15 or 30 seconds elicits little reflex tear secretion and so no anaesthetic is required to measure the basal secretion by this method (Hamano).

Tear drainage

Prior to tests of tear drainage, the lids, conjunctiva, and cornea should be examined to exclude disease that could account for excess tear production. The basic secretion test may also be appropriate as a deficiency may result in a reflex overproduction of tears. Syringing and dacrocystography are essential in evaluating epiphora. Dacroscintigraphy is of interest but is used little in practice. The primary dye test of Jones is used postoperatively to ascertain whether a patent channel exists between the eye and the nose.

Syringing
This can discriminate between a patent system, nasolacrimal duct block and canalicular block. Required equipment includes local anaesthetic, a punctal dilator, a syringe full of saline and a cannula.

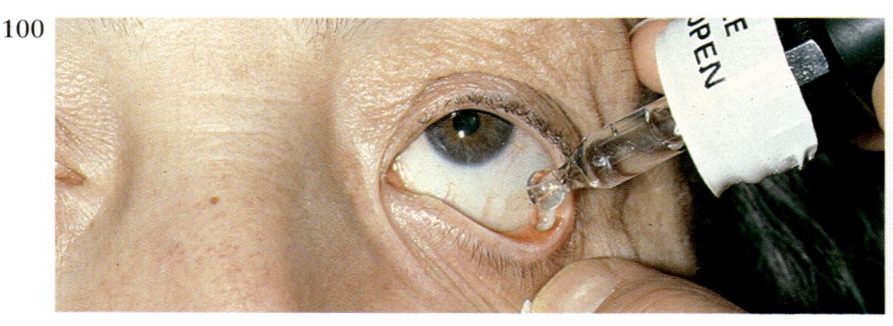

100 Syringing. The test can be performed with the patient seated or lying on a couch. Local anaesthetic drops are instilled.

101 Syringing. The lower punctum is dilated when the anaesthetic has taken effect.

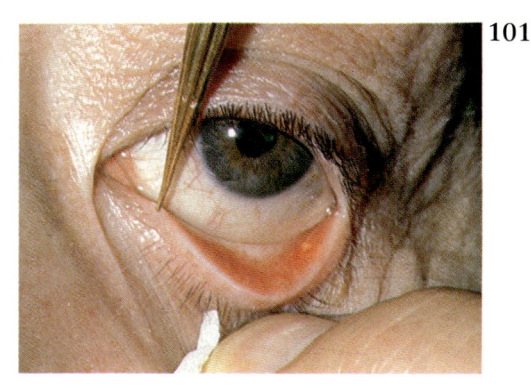

102 Syringing. The cannula is inserted into the dilated punctum, pointing downwards initially.

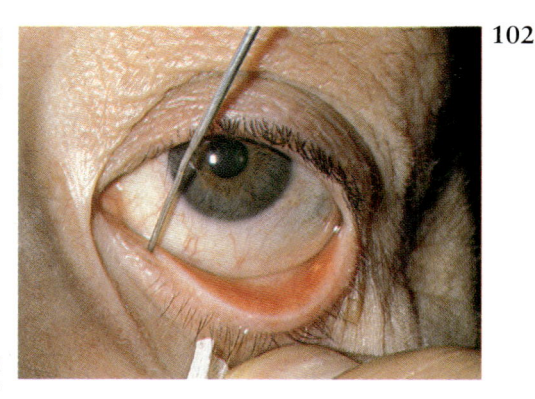

103 Syringing. The cannula is then angled medially to follow the course of the canaliculus while the lid is held laterally; if the canaliculi are clear, the cannula will pass through to meet the bony wall of the nose. If the canaliculus or common canaliculus is blocked a soft obstruction is felt. If the lid is not held laterally, the cannula will push the obstruction medially against the bony surface, and the examiner may think the cannula has entered the nasolacrimal sac.

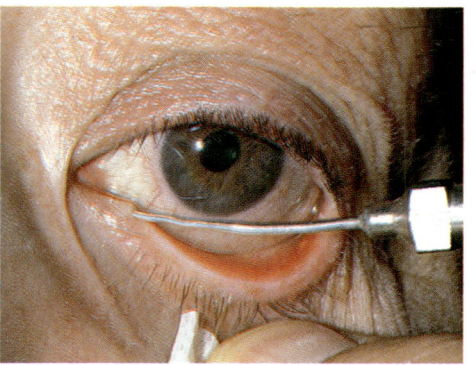

Saline is gently injected. If there is no obstruction, fluid will enter the patient's throat and he will mention that it tastes salty. Failure to notice fluid in the throat accompanied by regurgitation through the upper punctum demonstrates complete obstruction in the nasolacrimal duct or sac. If saline neither enters the nose nor flows back through the upper punctum, a canalicular obstruction is demonstrated. This method only identifies organic, not functional, blocks. The anatomy and nature of the block can be further defined by dacrocystography.

Dacrocystography (DCG)
This is performed in the radiology department. The practitioner wears protective shielding.

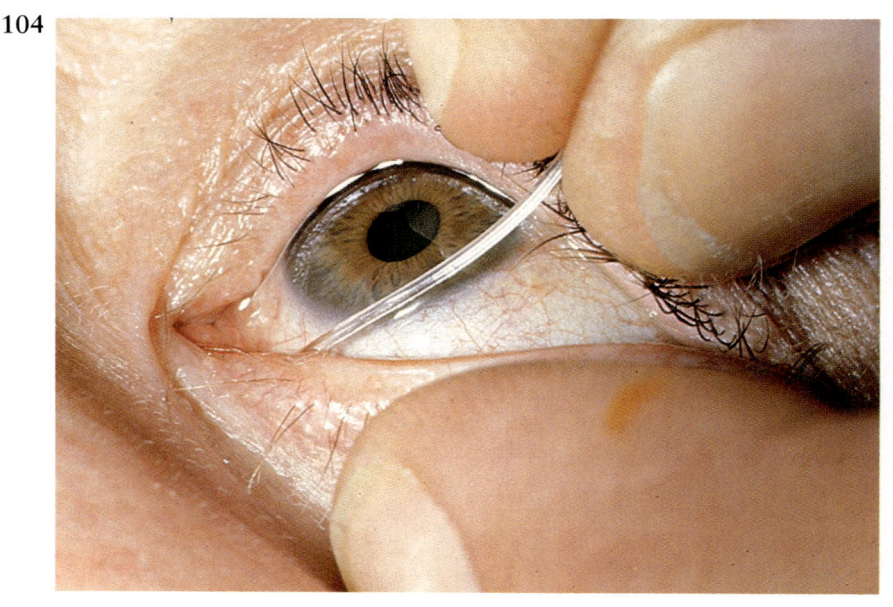

104 DCG. The technique is similar to syringing except that the puncta are intubated with polyethylene tubing so that the practitioner's hands are not in the field of the X-ray and bilateral injection can be performed simultaneously if required.

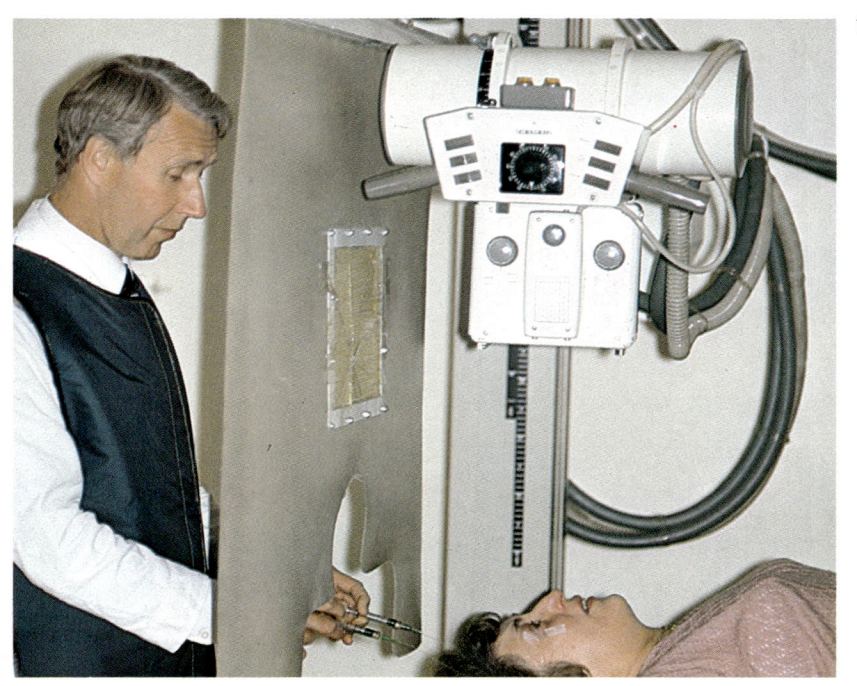

105 DCG. Radio-opaque contrast is injected. A plain film is taken initially then further films immediately following the contrast injection. X-rays taken under macro conditions provide a better view.

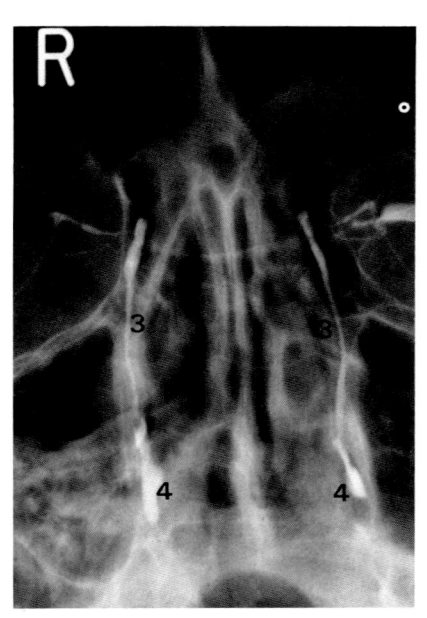

106 DCG. Contrast is seen in both eyes in the fornices (1), the canaliculi (2), common canaliculi, nasolacrimal ducts (3), and in the nose (4). This is a normal nasolacrimal system.

107 DCG. A right common canalicular block is present. Contrast has failed to enter the lacrimal sac and nasolacrimal duct. The left is normal.

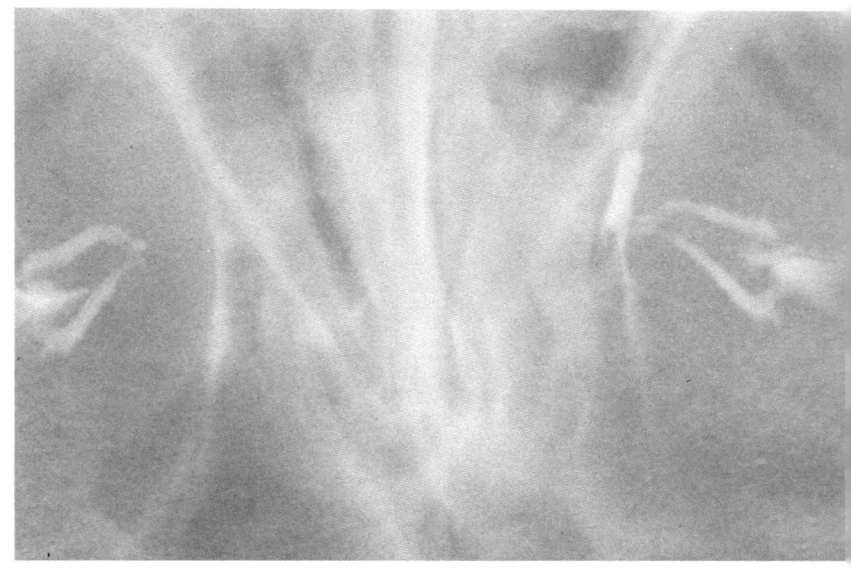

Jones' primary dye test

This is principally useful after surgery to ascertain whether a patent channel between the eye and the nose exists.

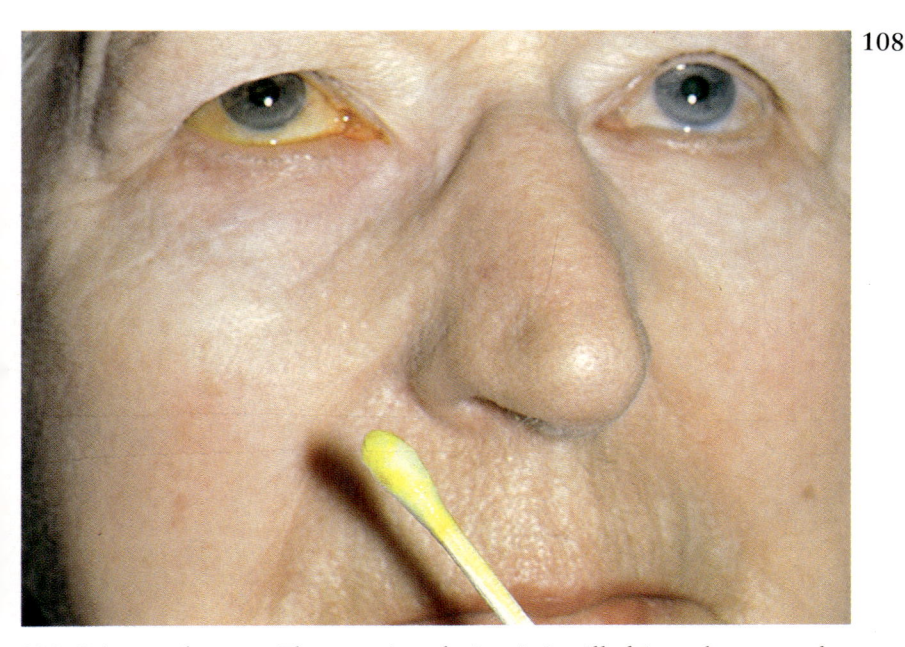

108 Primary dye test. Fluorescein solution is instilled into the eye and a cotton swab gently held up the same side of the nose under the anterior part of the inferior turbinate for a few minutes. The appearance of dye on the swab, which may be enhanced by blue light, confirms a clear passage.

7 Use of the slit-lamp

The slit-lamp (biomicroscope) provides a magnified, stereoscopic view of anterior ocular structures. A variable illumination system and a binocular microscope with a fixed focal plane are mounted on a movable base plate, and the whole is elevated on a stand. The anterior chamber angle, posterior vitreous, and fundus can be examined using accessory lenses (Chapters 9 and 10).

The patient is seated at the instrument which is adjusted to a suitable height. He places his chin on the chin rest and his forehead against the bar.

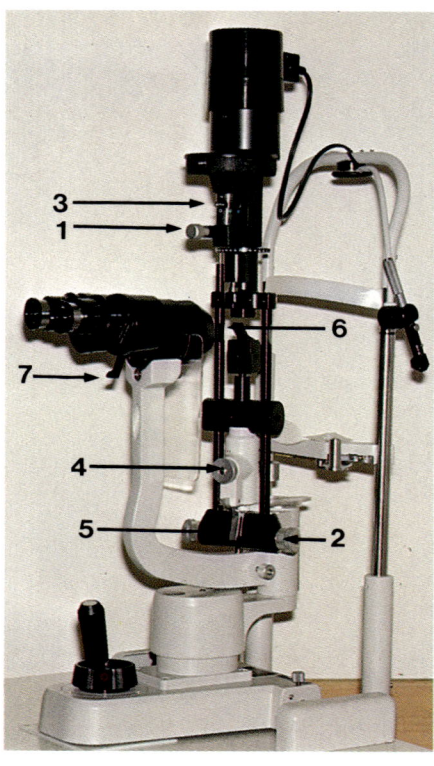

109 The slit-lamp. The illumination adjustments are the height (1) and width (2) of the beam (with associated scales for measurement of anterior segment structures), and the use of additional filters (3). These include an infra-red filter, used for most examinations, a neutral density filter, to decrease the light intensity, a red-free (green) filter to enhance the view when red objects are examined, and a blue filter, used when fluorescein has been instilled into the eye. The beam can be displaced laterally (4) to avoid directly illuminating the object in focus (see **117, 118**), or tilted upwards (5) when oblique or horizontal for an optimal view of the vitreous. The standard mirror (6) can be replaced with a short mirror for contact lens fundus examination. There are two magnification settings (7).

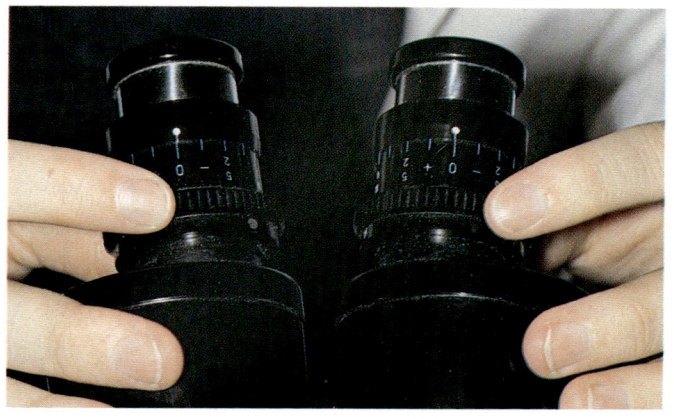

110 The eyepieces. These can be adjusted for myopic or hypermetropic examiners and the emmetrope should check that they are on the 0 setting prior to use. Spectacles can be worn while using the slit-lamp if necessary. The examiner adjusts the interpupillary distance of the eyepieces to suit him. Looking through the eyepieces, the examiner moves the base of the slit-lamp towards the patient to bring the eye into focus.

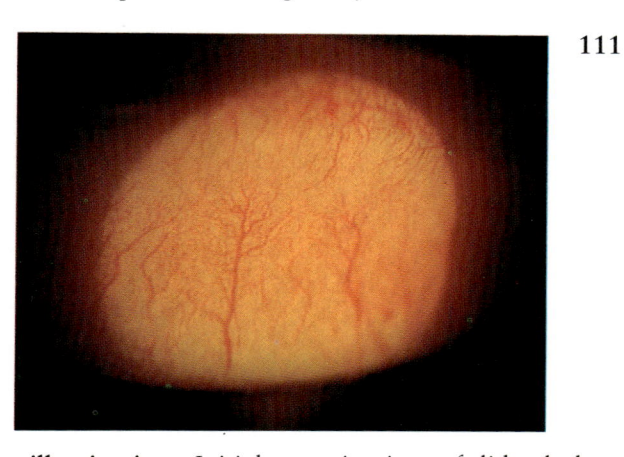

111 Diffuse illumination. Initial examination of lids, lashes, tarsal conjunctiva (with everted lid), bulbar conjunctiva, cornea and iris is performed with a dim light so as not to dazzle the patient, a tall broad beam, and low magnification. This provides a view of the surface of the structure examined. The upper tarsal conjunctiva is shown.

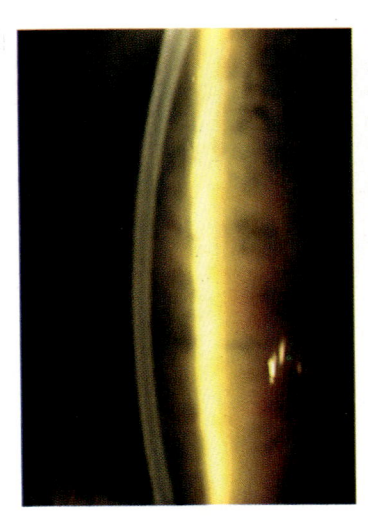

112 Direct illumination. The cornea and anterior chamber (and lens and anterior vitreous if pupil dilatation permits) can then be viewed with a bright light, narrow beam and high magnification. This provides a cross-sectional view of the structures, revealing the different layers and their approximate thickness. The cornea is shown.

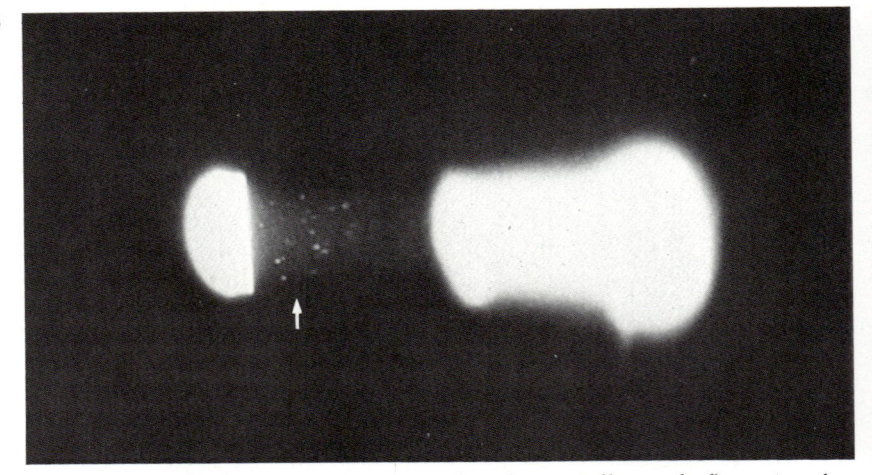

113 Direct illumination—anterior chamber. Cells and flare in the anterior chamber can be seen clearly with the brightest light, a short narrow beam (a spotlight), and high magnification. The examiner looks at the beam in the area before the pupil where the cells stand out brightly against the black background (arrow). Careful focussing may be necessary to see them. The anterior vitreous is examined in the same way, focussing behind the lens, through a dilated pupil.

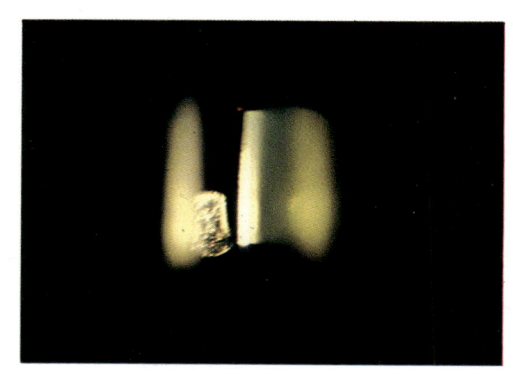

114 Direct illumination—the lens. The lens can be seen in cross-section without dilatation using the bright light and short narrow beam directed through the pupil.

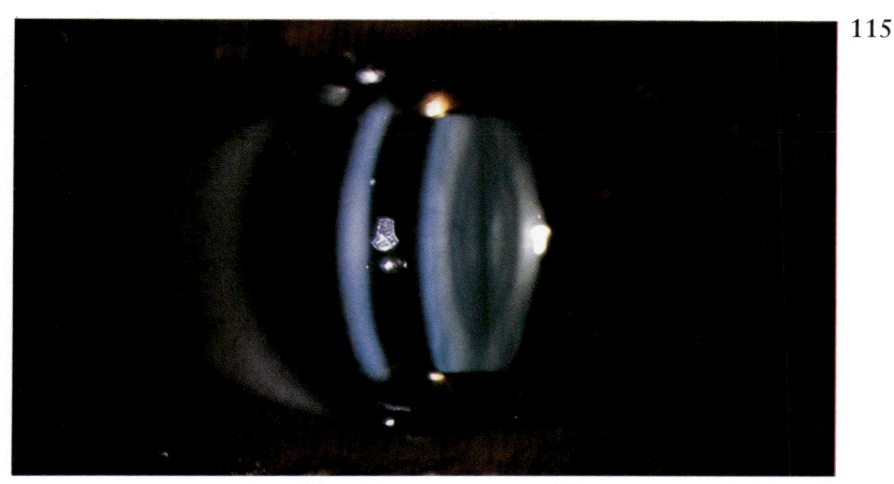

115 Direct illumination—the lens. It is best examined after dilatation. This is a normal lens.

Three other techniques are used: retroillumination (reflected illumination), sclerotic scatter (indirect lateral illumination) and specular reflection.

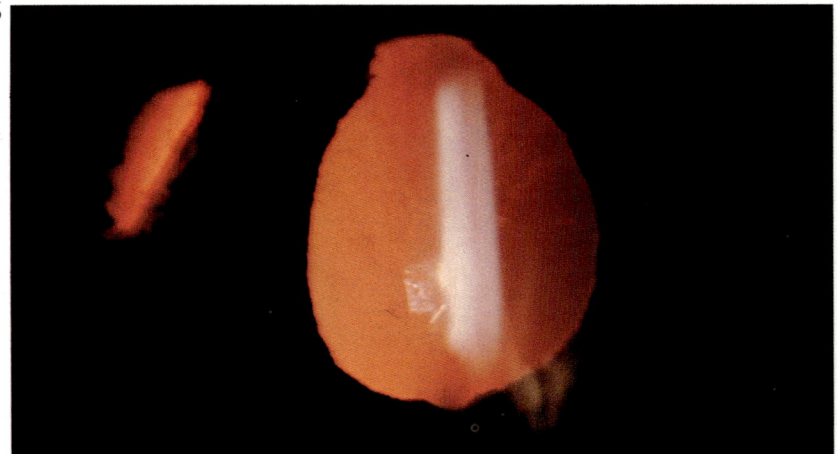

116 Retroillumination—iris dialysis. In retroillumination the area is lit by diffuse reflection from tissues behind it. Here the beam is aligned axially and reduced to a size smaller than the pupil. Directing the light through the pupil produces a red reflex which shows up defects in the iris and is particularly helpful in suspected intra-ocular foreign bodies where the iris has been penetrated.

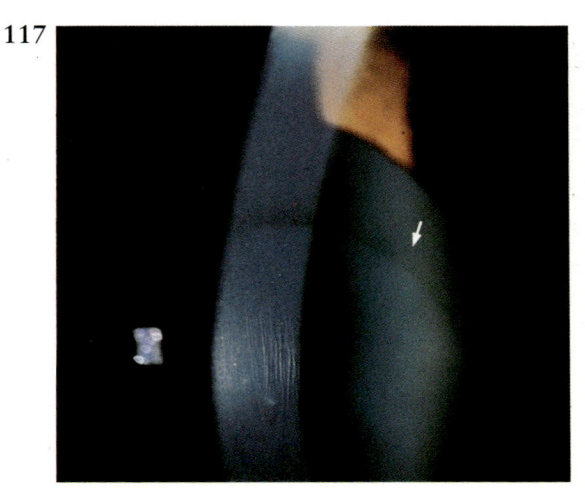

117 Retroillumination—keratoconus. The beam can also be displaced laterally to illuminate the cornea with light reflected from the iris or lens. Here a Fleischer iron ring is seen in reflected light (arrow). (Vertical stress lines are also visible at the corneal apex.)

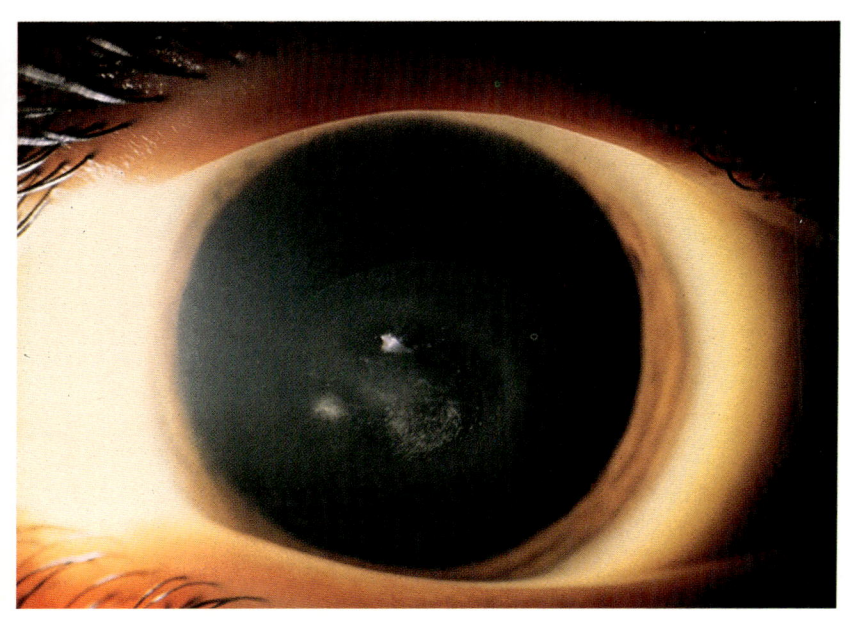

118 Sclerotic scatter—keratoconus. The beam is again displaced laterally by loosening the illumination centration screw, so that light falls on the limbus while the examiner focusses on the cornea, and light reflected within the cornea illuminates early corneal oedema or fine corneal opacities. This technique is also used for other structures when it is termed indirect lateral illumination; the beam is aimed at a point beside the object in focus which is illuminated by stray light.

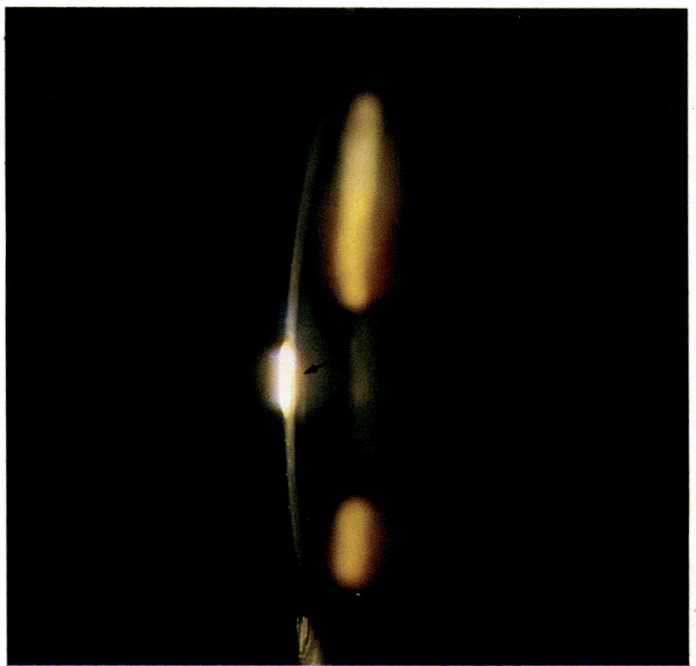

119 Specular reflection. The endothelium can be examined by this means. The beam and viewing system are locked at 20° to 30° to each other. The posterior cornea is brought into focus, and the locked beam and microscope are rotated about the vertical axis until a bright reflex is seen as shown. The bright reflex is from the corneal epithelial surface. A small amount of light is reflected from the endothelium in the area adjacent to the bright reflection (arrow). The cell mosaic is visible there when observed with high magnification and careful focussing because the intercellular matrix reflects light at different angles to the cell bodies.

8 Tests relevant to the conjunctiva, cornea and anterior chamber

Use of fluorescein

Fluorescence occurs when a substance emits light of a certain wavelength after being excited by light of a different wavelength. Sodium fluorescein is water soluble and emits light of a wavelength approximately 520 nm (green) after receiving light of approximately 490 nm (blue). Concentrations from 0.25 to 2 per cent are used on the cornea.

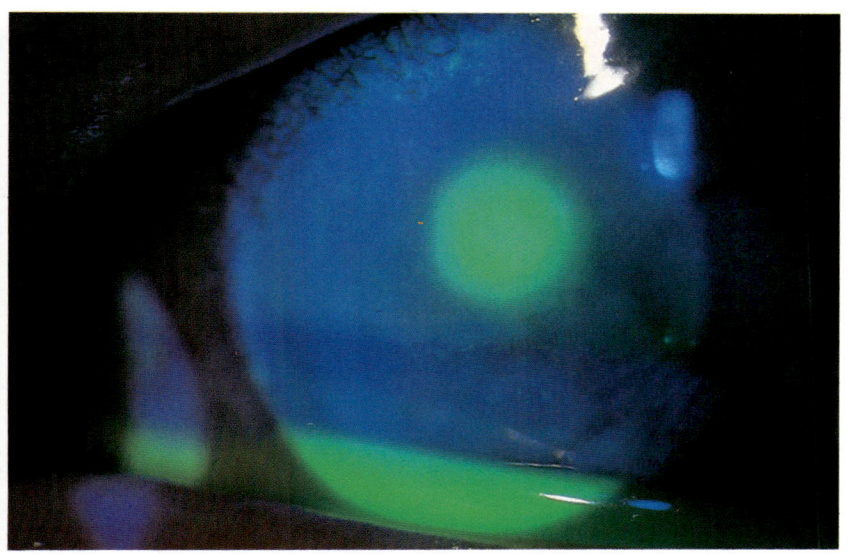

120 Fluorescein. Fluorescein stains defects in the corneal epithelium. An ulcer is shown fluorescing green under blue light.

Fluorescein is also used for applanation tonometry (Chapter 9), fluorescein angiography (Chapter 10) and Seidel's test (Chapter 11).

Use of rose bengal

Rose bengal is a water-soluble dye which stains mucin and devitalized cells. It is uncomfortable for the patient and is best applied in small quantities to the superior bulbar conjunctiva (to be spread over the cornea during blinking), or after local anaesthetic. A 1 per cent concentration is commonly used.

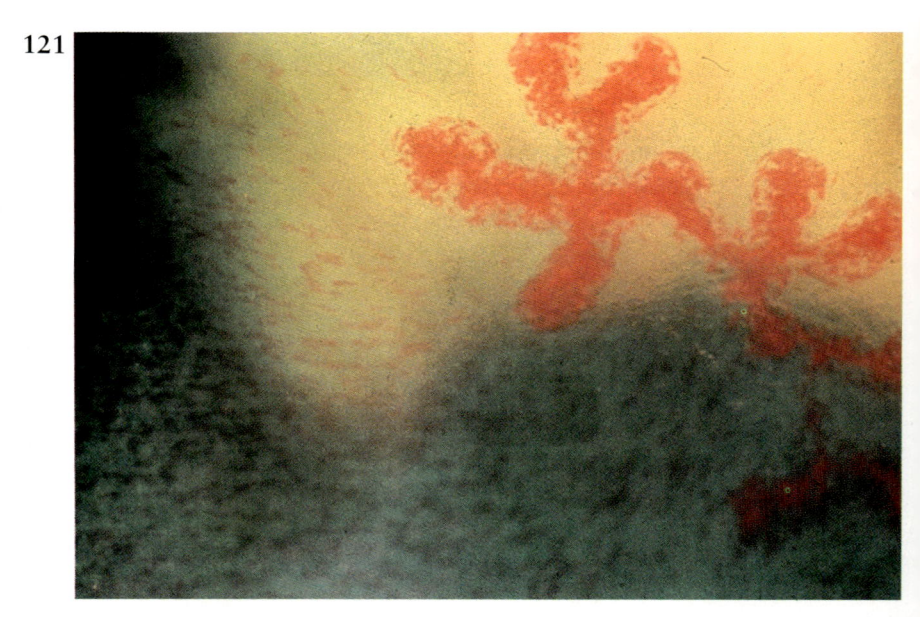

121 Rose bengal. A dendritic ulcer takes up rose bengal into the infected cells bordering the ulcer.

Microbiology

The notification of the laboratory and immediate transport and examination of specimens is as important as obtaining material, to avoid drying and deterioration of the samples.

Conjunctival swab
In suspected bacterial conjunctivitis, or in corneal ulcers, a conjunctival swab is routinely performed.

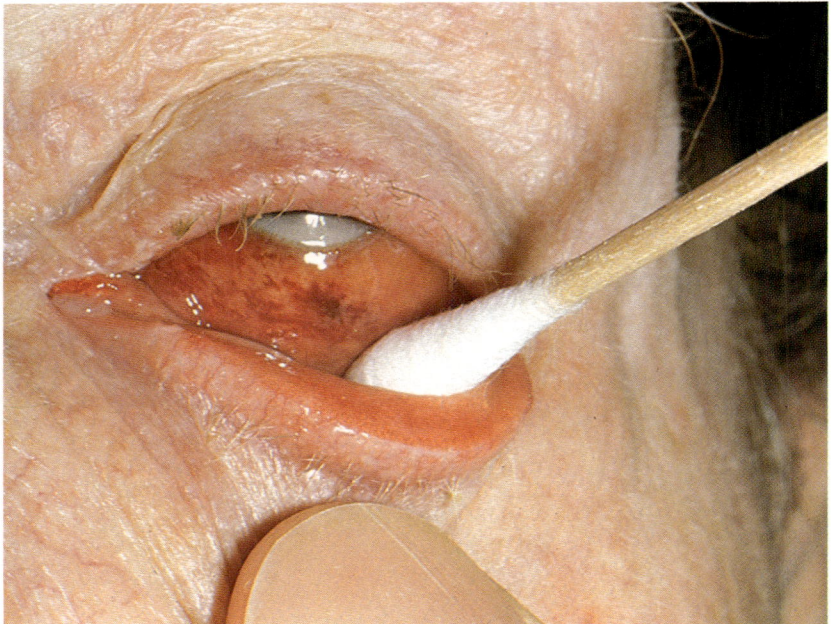

122 Conjunctival swab. A sterile cotton bud is moistened with sterile saline and swept across the palpebral conjunctiva of the lower lid, avoiding the skin and eyelashes. This is plated out onto blood agar at once.

If the conjunctivitis is purulent, a second fresh swab is taken and spread onto a clean glass slide for Gram staining. If it is not purulent, there is not usually enough material to produce a helpful result on Gram stain.

Conjunctival scraping

Conjunctival scraping is performed by scraping the anaesthetized tarsal conjunctival epithelium with a sterile metal spatula, and spreading the material onto a clean glass slide for Giemsa staining. This technique is of importance in diagnosis of chlamydial infection. A Dacron swab used in this context provides material for immunofluorescence and chlamydial culture.

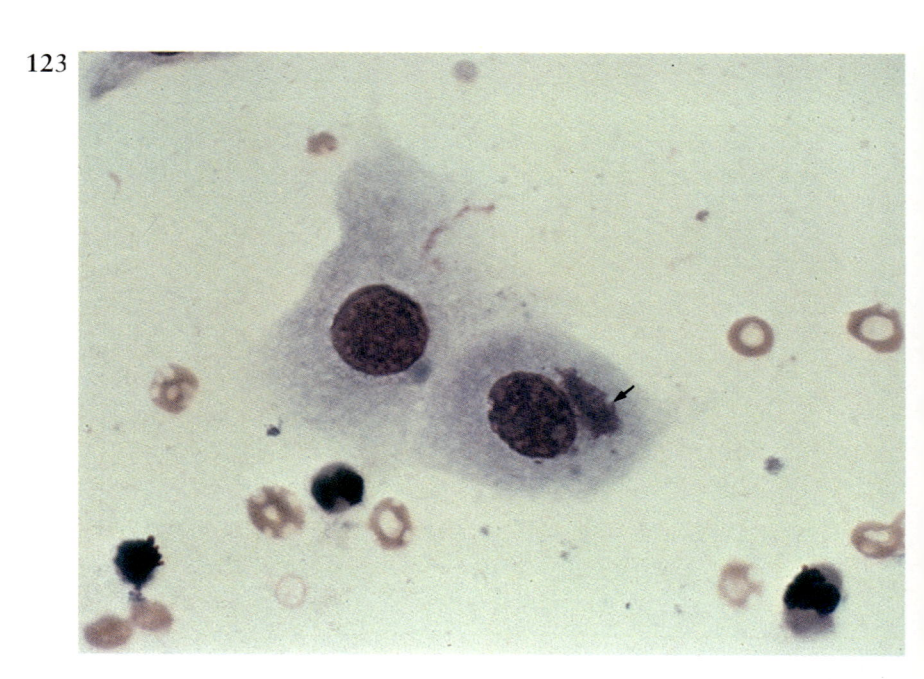

123 Giemsa stain. Giemsa staining demonstrates chlamydial inclusions (arrow) in conjunctival cells.

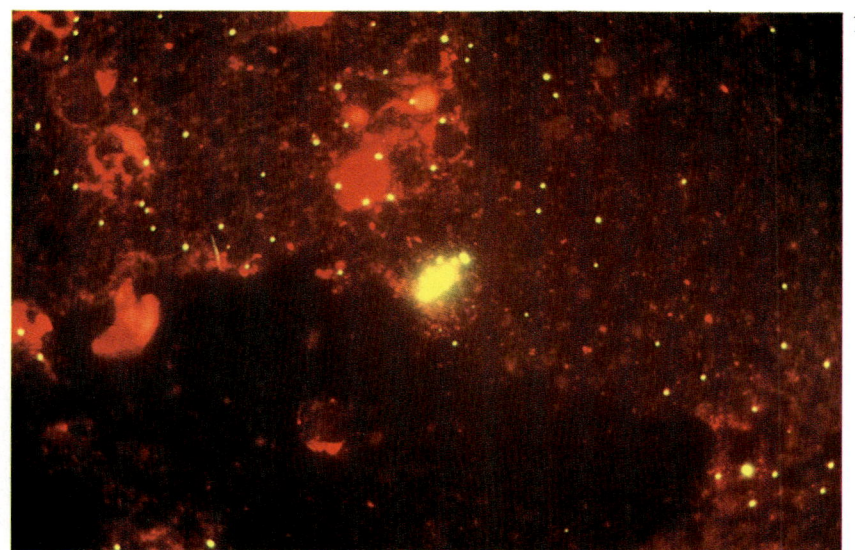

124 Immunofluorescence. Chlamydial infection is more reliably demonstrated by immunofluorescent staining techniques. Multiple small fluorescing dots (elementary bodies) and a large central inclusion are seen in conjunctival cells above.

Corneal scraping

Ulcers other than the obviously dendritic are scraped under slit-lamp magnification to obtain material for microbiological diagnosis. It is often recommended that material be plated onto a number of different media but in practice it is difficult to obtain enough for more than one plate and possibly for a Gram stain. Therefore the first scraping is spread on blood agar which is readily available and suitable for common outer eye bacterial pathogens, except *Haemophilus* and *Neisseria* species which require chocolate agar. Among fungi, most Candida organisms (yeasts) will also grow on blood agar. A second scraping is then taken for Gram stain, smeared on a clean glass slide, and stained and examined at once by an experienced microbiologist.

Growth failure is more likely to be due to a poor specimen or previous antibiotics than an inappropriate medium. If an ulcer is improving on an antibiotic regimen there is no need to repeat the scraping, but if it is static or deteriorating a repeat scraping is then performed for growth on special media, e.g. Sabouraud's (fungi), after discussion with the microbiologist.

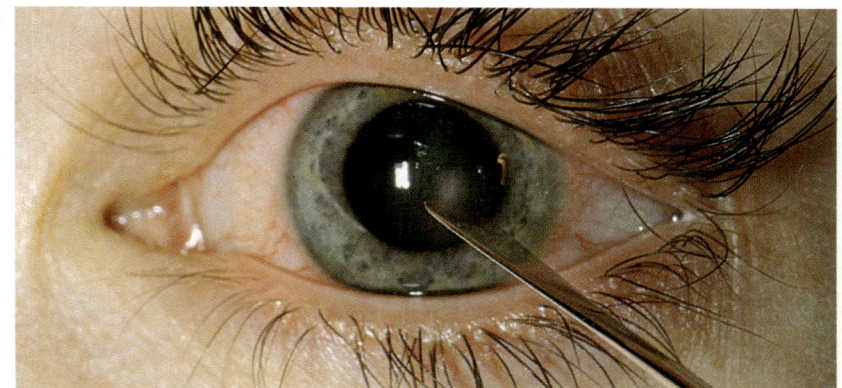

125 Corneal scraping. The procedure may be painful so the eye is anaesthetized, though preservatives in local anaesthetic preparations may inhibit bacterial growth. A sterile metal spatula or wire loop is used to scrape the centre and margins of the ulcer under slit-lamp observation, avoiding contact with the eyelids.

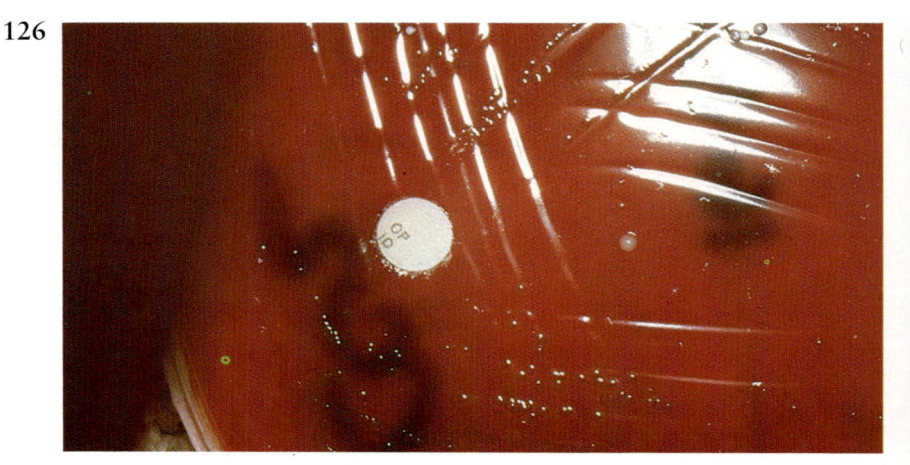

126 Corneal scraping. The material is then spread on a fresh agar plate, either in C streaks or zigzags. This is to dilute the bacterial matter so that growth in single colonies will occur in the latter part of the pattern. The spatula should not be buried in the agar but should slide across it.

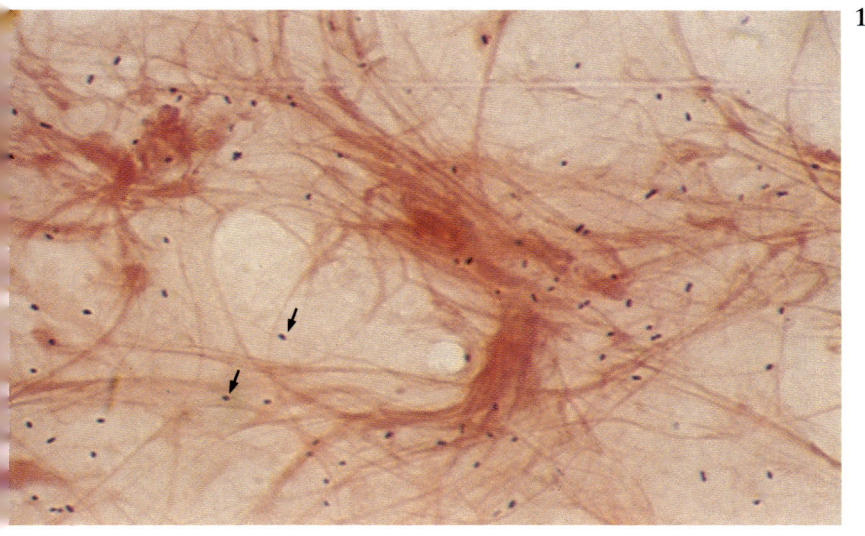

127 Gram stain. *Pneumococcus* (Gram positive).

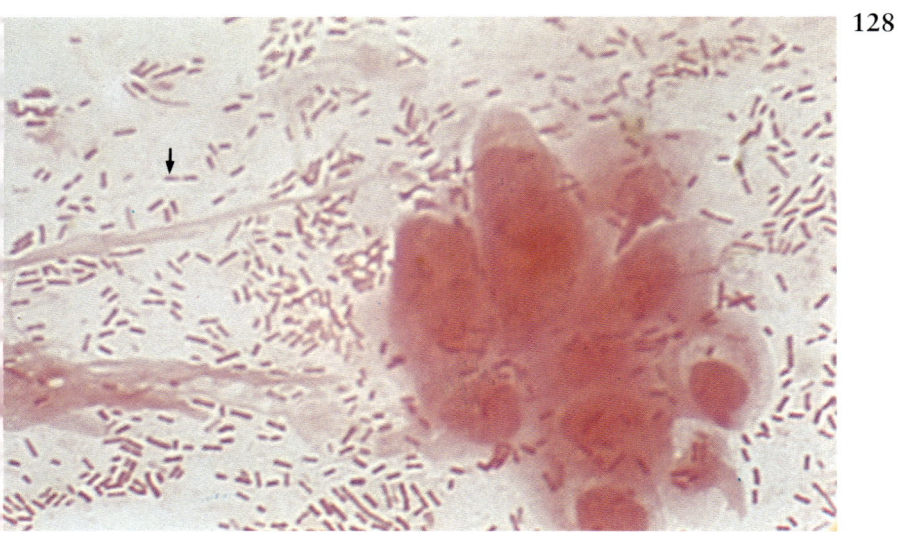

128 Gram stain. *Moraxella* (Gram negative).

Specular microscopy

The formal investigation of the corneal endothelium requires a specular microscope which is an instrument incorporating corneal magnification, appropriate illumination, and a camera to record the endothelial appearance for subsequent analysis. (Specular reflection with the slit-lamp has been described in Chapter 7.)

129 Specular microscopy. An objective lens on the head of the microscope in contact with the patient's cornea permits viewing and photography.

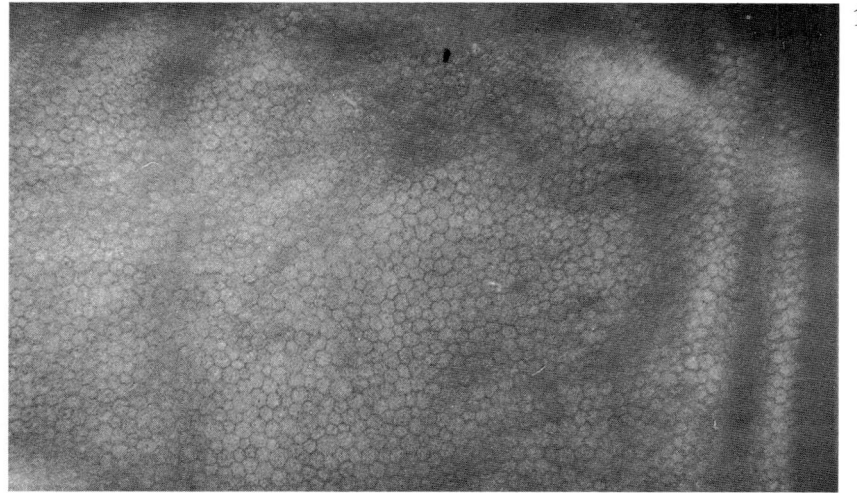

130 Specular microscopy. An example of the resulting photographic record. Normal endothelium.

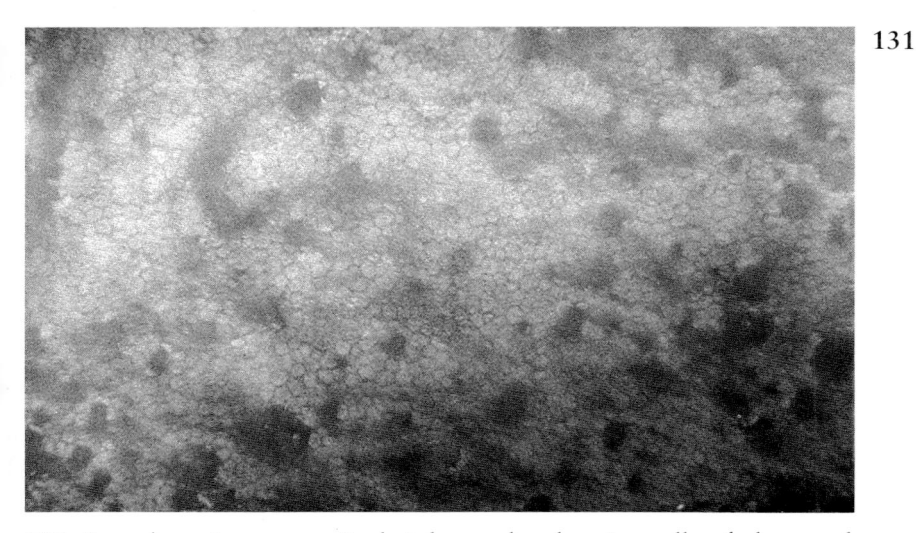

131 Specular microscopy. Fuchs' dystrophy showing cells of abnormal size and shape and excrescences.

Pachymetry

The thickness of the cornea or of the anterior chamber can be measured using a pachymeter, for example to assess endothelial function or where closed-angle glaucoma is suspected. This instrument uses an image splitter consisting of two plano plates of glass, one above the other, in which the upper plate can be rotated to move the upper part of the image. Ultrasonic pachymetry is also available.

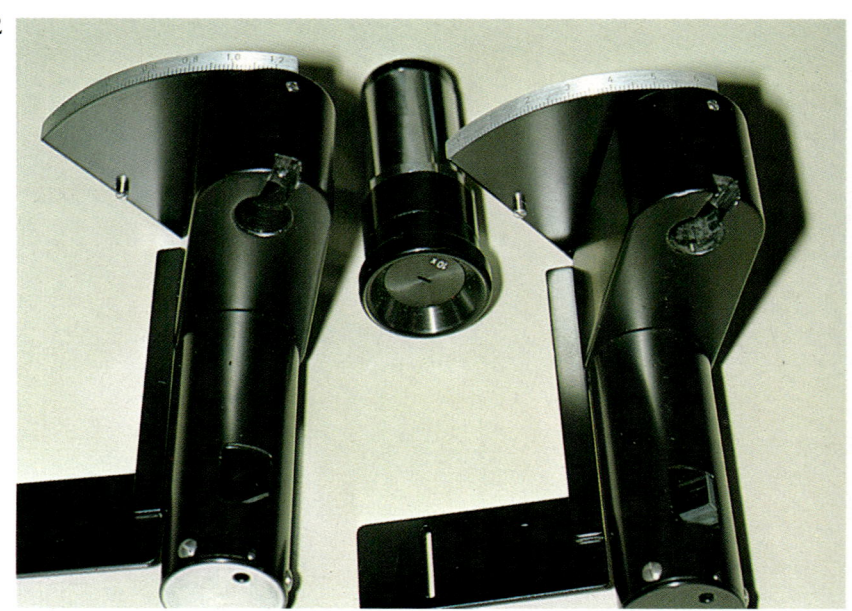

132 Pachymetry. Measuring devices with different calibration are used for the cornea and anterior chamber.

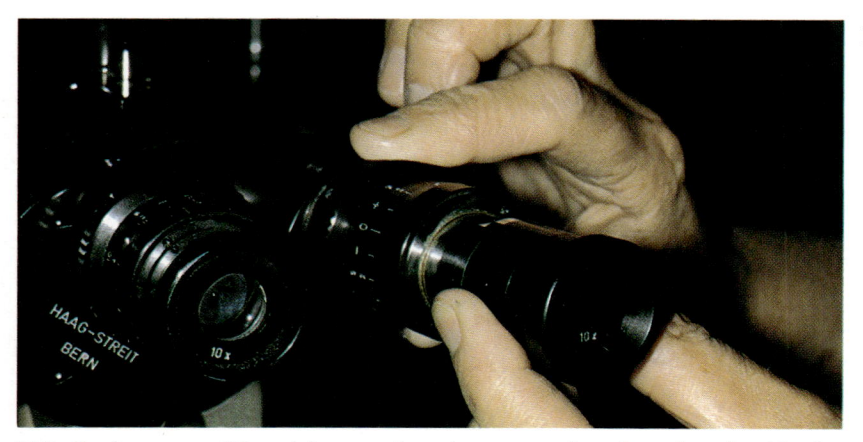

133 Pachymetry. The right eyepiece is removed and replaced with the 10 x split image eyepiece rotated until the split is horizontal. For corneal pachymetry the eyepiece is adjusted to +2.5 dioptres, for anterior chamber pachymetry to +6 dioptres.

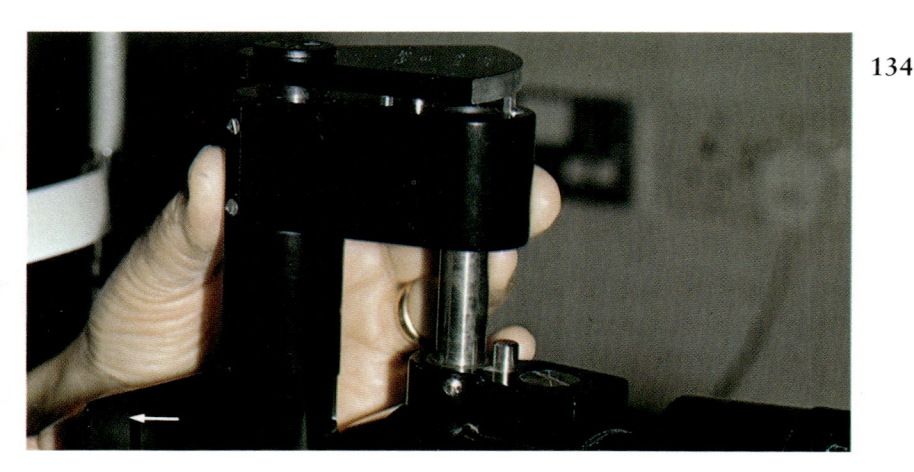

134 Pachymetry. The appropriate measuring device is run onto the fixation base attached to the microscope body. The beam is rotated until it passes through the vertical opening of the measuring device (arrow) and fixed at that angle of 40°. The whole is then rotated until the beam is directed at right angles to the corneal surface at the pupil centre.

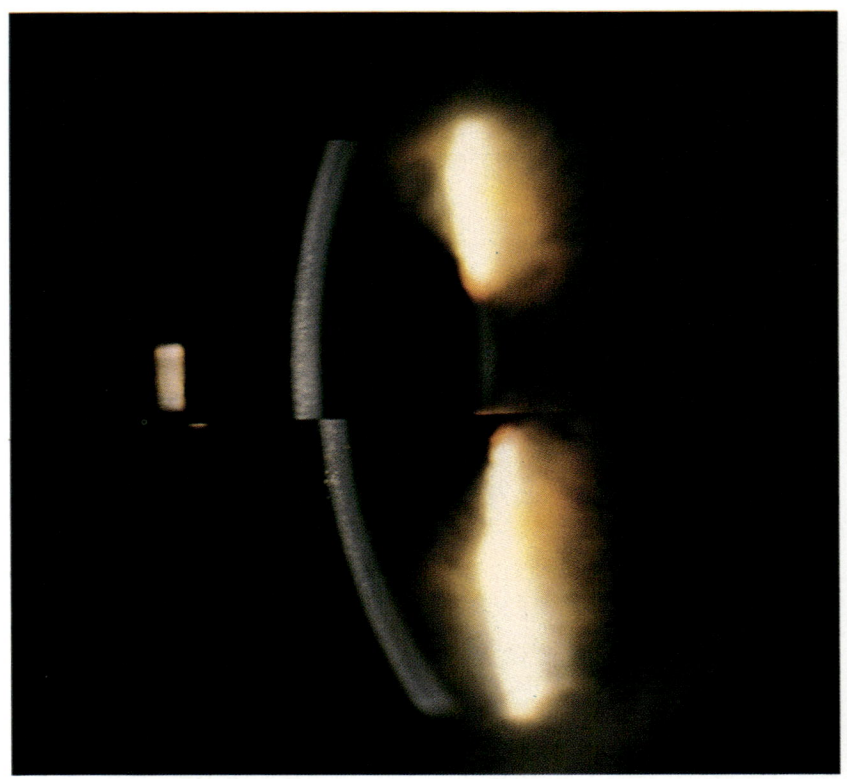

135 Pachymetry. The joystick is adjusted until the cornea (or anterior chamber) is in the middle of the field. The scale is then rotated so that the upper glass plate moves through the distance to be measured: for the cornea, the endothelium in the upper image is made to coincide with the epithelium in the lower image; for the anterior chamber depth, the anterior surface of the lens above is made to coincide with the corneal epithelium below, and the corneal thickness is then subtracted.

9 Tests in glaucoma

Tonometry

The applanation tonometer (Goldmann) is used for all routine testing of the intra-ocular pressure. The indentation tonometer (Schiotz) should not be used if applanation is available as it is less accurate. 'Digital tonometry', i.e. finger pressure on the globe, is unacceptable as a means of measuring intra-ocular pressure accurately, although gross changes may be identified.

If the cornea is irregular or deformed by disease, a reading can still often be obtained by careful applanation in the more normal area without recourse to other instruments.

Applanation tonometry—Goldmann

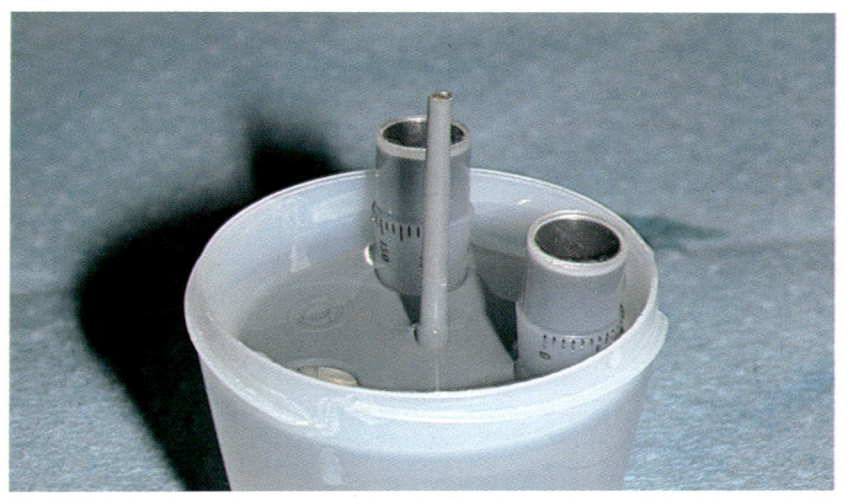

136 Disinfection of tonometer heads. Fresh solutions of 1:10 household bleach (5000 ppm of available chlorine) or 3 per cent hydrogen peroxide have been recommended. Ten minutes of soaking should ensure disinfection. The head should be rinsed prior to use.

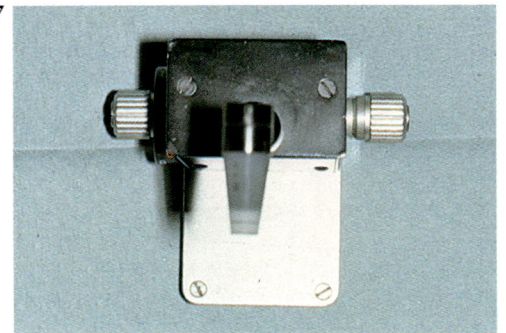

137 Tonometry. The prism is removed from solution, rinsed, dried and inserted into the bracket so that the split in the prism is horizontal. The prism is aligned with the tonometer; it will settle into a slot when it is straight.

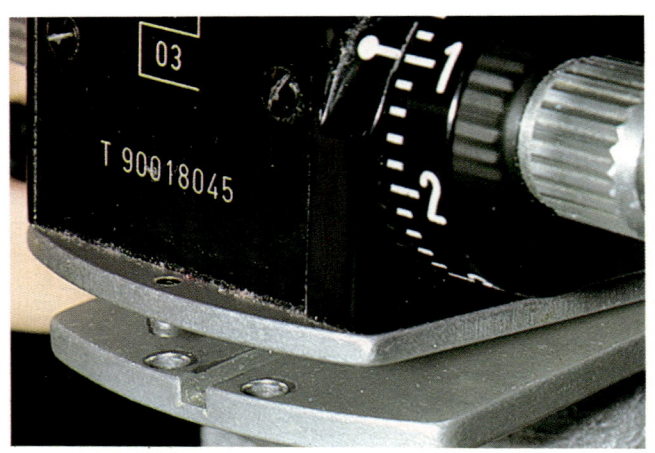

138 Tonometry. The tonometer is inserted into its support on the slit-lamp. Note that the stud is not put into the central groove, but into either the right pit or the left one. The instrument is used monocularly and if it is inserted into the left pit, the left eyepiece is used. In some models the tonometer is swung over from the side or above and should settle in the correct position. The scale on the side of the tonometer is adjusted to read between 10 and 20 mm Hg.

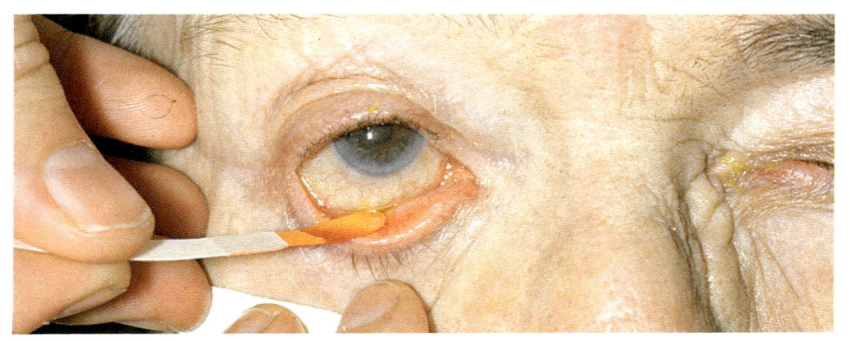

139 Tonometry. The best means of application of fluorescein for tonometry is with a sterile impregnated strip. This is moistened with sterile water, saline, or local anaesthetic and dabbed into the lower fornix. If fluorescein solutions or dye/local anaesthetic mixtures in bottles are used, they need to be changed daily to avoid bacterial contamination e.g. by Pseudomonas. A weak local anaesthetic, e.g. benoxinate hydrochloride 0.4 per cent, may be added separately.

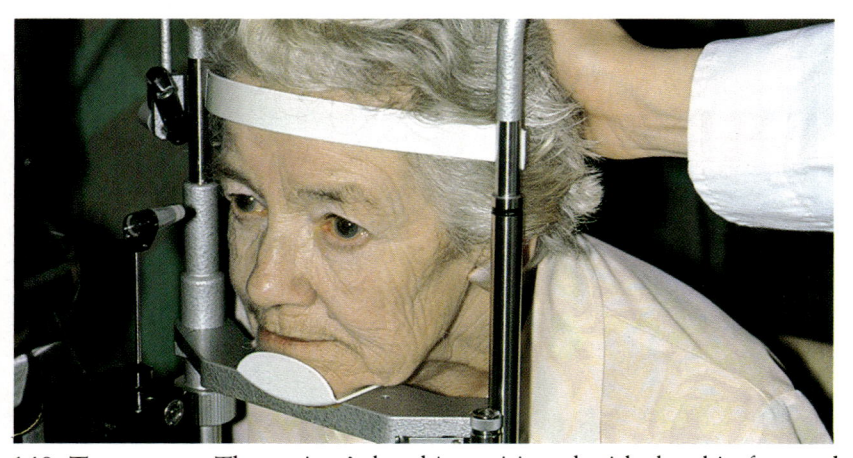

140 Tonometry. The patient's head is positioned with the chin forward in the chin rest and the forehead against the bar. An assistant may hold the head gently in position if the patient is inclined to move back. The illumination beam should be broad and at about 60° to the microscope for best illumination. The blue filter is used.

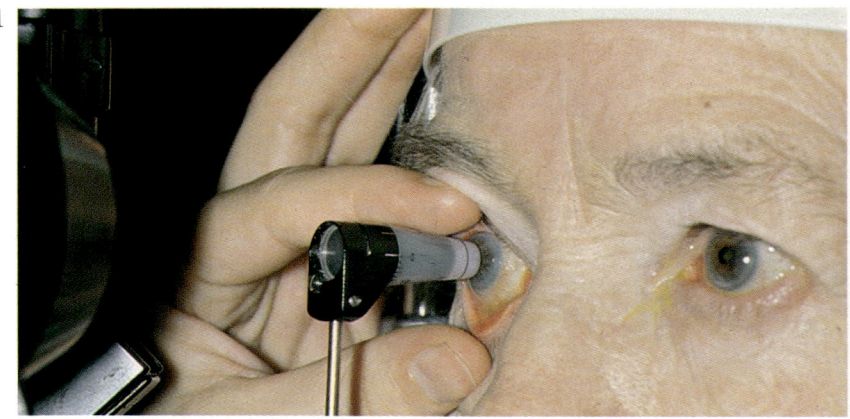

141 Tonometry. The tonometer is pushed towards the eye by advancing the entire base plate of the slit-lamp. The fine control joystick is held back. Then, using the latter, the prism tip is gently advanced onto the cornea under direct vision. Patients commonly blink or move as the prism approaches and the eye may be held open in a way similar to that described for gonioscopy, making sure any pressure is upwards to the orbital rim rather than back to the globe.

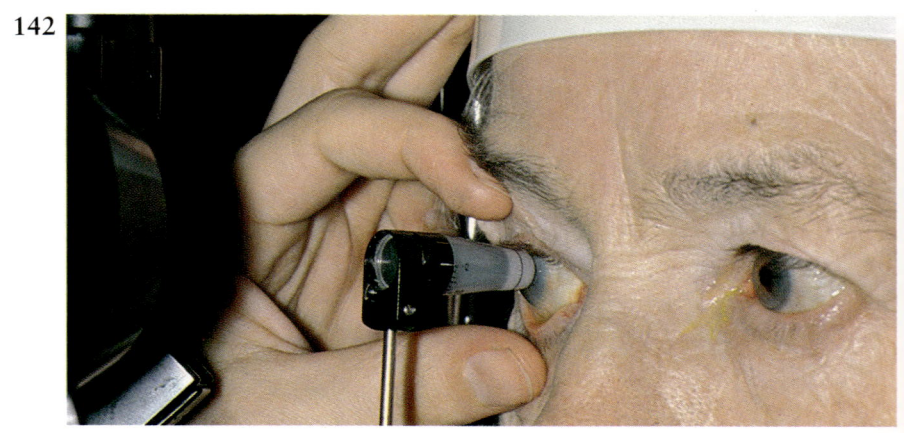

142 Tonometry. Holding the lid incorrectly may allow it to fall onto the prism.

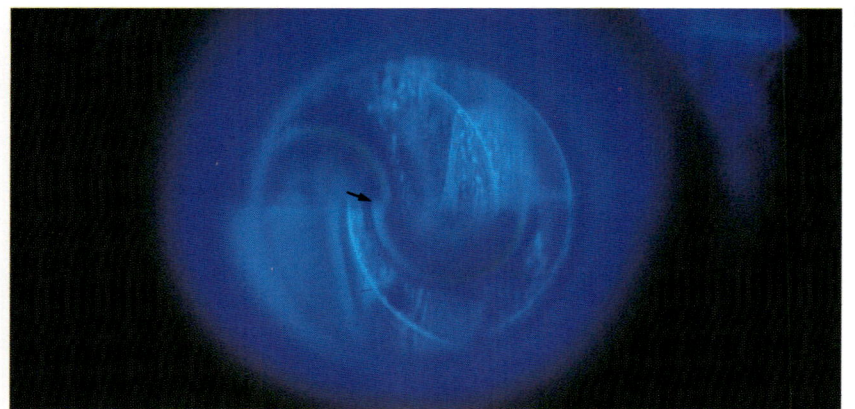

143 Tonometry. The examiner looks through the appropriate eyepiece. The correct endpoint is seen above; the inner borders of each green fluorescein crescent must overlap (arrow). The ring represents fluorescein pushed to the periphery of the contact zone, i.e. the inner border of the ring surrounds the area flattened by contact. The scale on the right of the tonometer is adjusted to achieve the endpoint. The reading multiplied by 10 is the intra-ocular pressure in mm Hg. The instrument is removed from the eye.

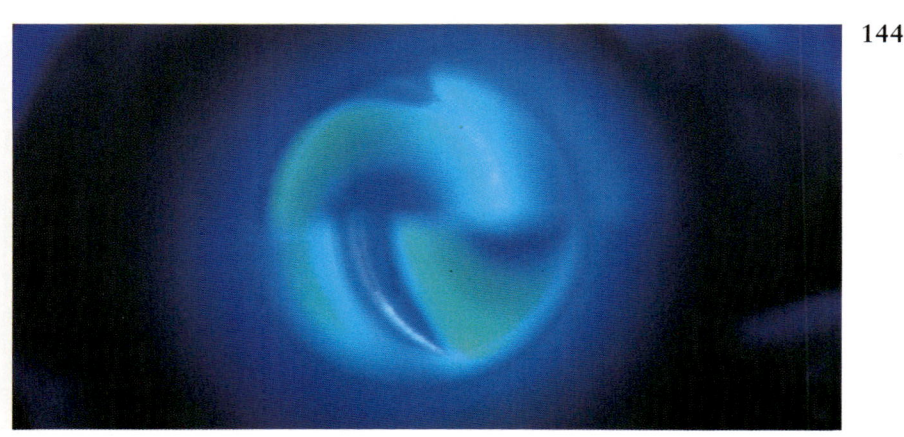

144 Tonometry. The endpoint as seen with thicker crescents. It is preferable to wipe the prism and repeat.

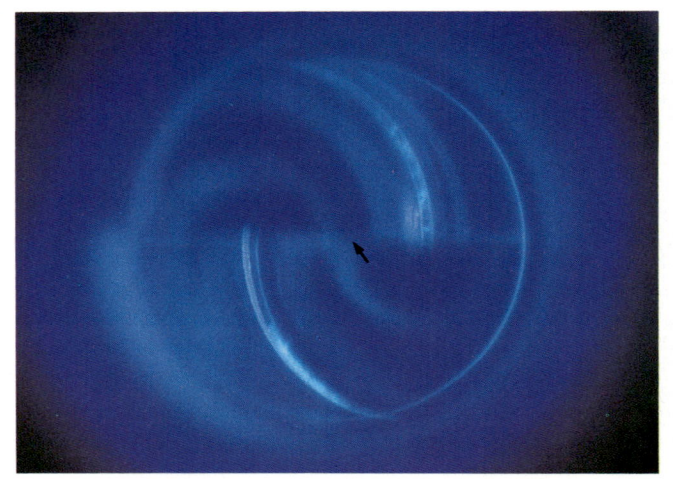

145 Tonometry. The crescents are not overlapping sufficiently (arrow); this is not the correct endpoint.

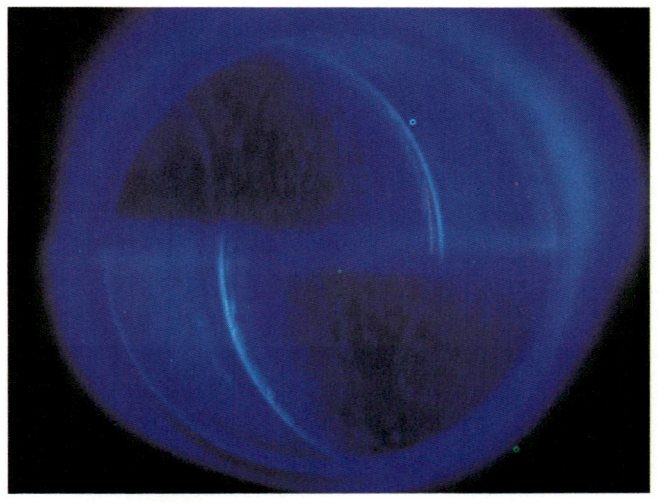

146 Tonometry. The prism is not on the eye; the patient may have moved backwards. These bright crescents are part of the applanating head itself.

If the rings overlap markedly and do not move with movement of the scale, the tonometer is pressing too hard on the cornea. It must be withdrawn and correctly repositioned.

Applanation tonometry—Perkins
This instrument allows applanation tonometry when a slit-lamp is unavailable or a patient must remain supine.

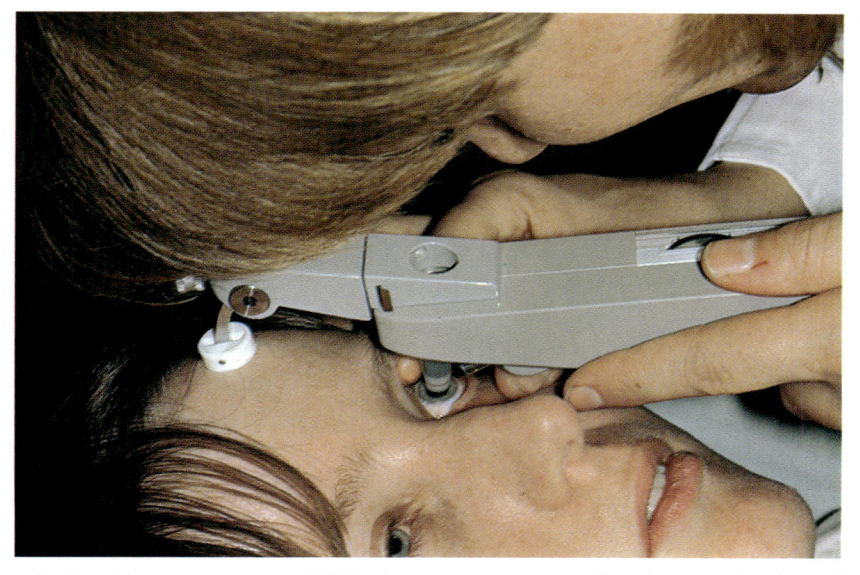

147 Perkins tonometry. With the patient supine, local anaesthetic and fluorescein are instilled as usual. The prism is inserted into the holder of the Perkins tonometer. The lids are held apart and the prism gently placed on the cornea while the examiner looks through the viewing aperture. The scale on the side of the handle is adjusted with the thumb of the hand holding the tonometer to the same endpoint as for Goldmann tonometry.

Visual field testing

Important variables are the angular subtense (degrees) of field examined, the distance from the subject (and hence the size of the defects discovered), whether the target moves (kinetic perimetry) or is static (static perimetry) and whether the threshold is tested or a supraliminal stimulus is used. A cooperative patient and an interpreting examiner are required for both the tangent screen (Bjerrum screen) and Goldmann perimetry. The Friedmann analyser can be operated reliably after a brief training and relies somewhat less on patient compliance. Automated perimeters are used increasingly but the principles of manual perimetry should still be understood.

Tangent screen
Available screens vary in size. They are designed to examine the central 30° of visual field at either 1 or 2 metres. Targets on the end of black wands against a black screen have traditionally been used. An alternative is a focussed light, directed at the screen from behind the patient.

148 Tangent screen. The patient sits 2 m away from the screen, wearing a lens correction for distance if necessary. One eye is occluded. He is asked to observe the central marker, and not follow the target. A large cross of white tape will help to indicate it if his acuity is poor.

The test is explained: a target will be shown on the screen and the patient, while constantly viewing the central marker, should report when he is aware of the target in his field of vision. The examiner brings the test target in from the periphery in several parts of each quadrant. He notes where the target is seen, paying particular attention to points on either side of the vertical and horizontal meridia, in case of neuro-ophthalmological lesions, or a nasal step in glaucoma.

The central area is checked for scotomas by showing the target briefly at various points in the central 20°. If the patient does not see the target, the defect is mapped out by moving the test object from the blind to the seeing area in several directions. The same procedure is used for the blind spot, initially placing the target between 10° and 15° in the lateral horizontal meridian where the blind spot is approximately located.

148

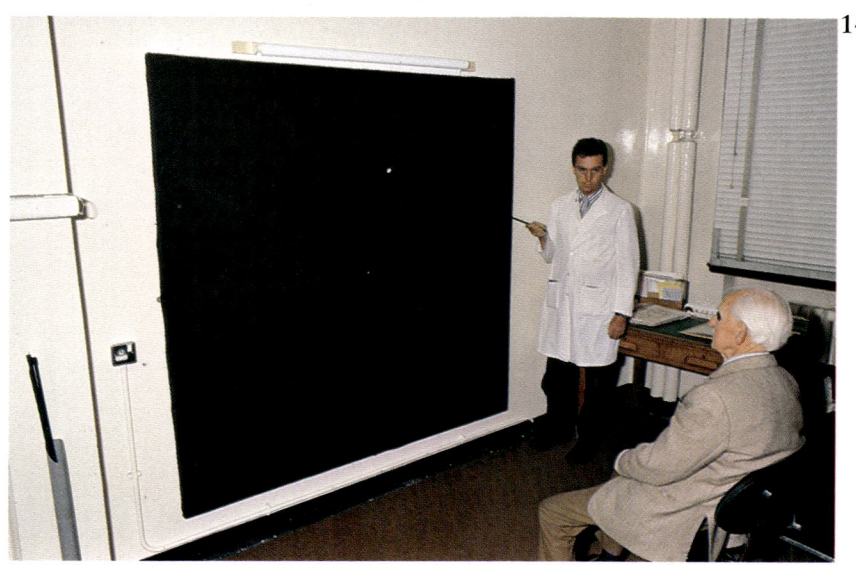

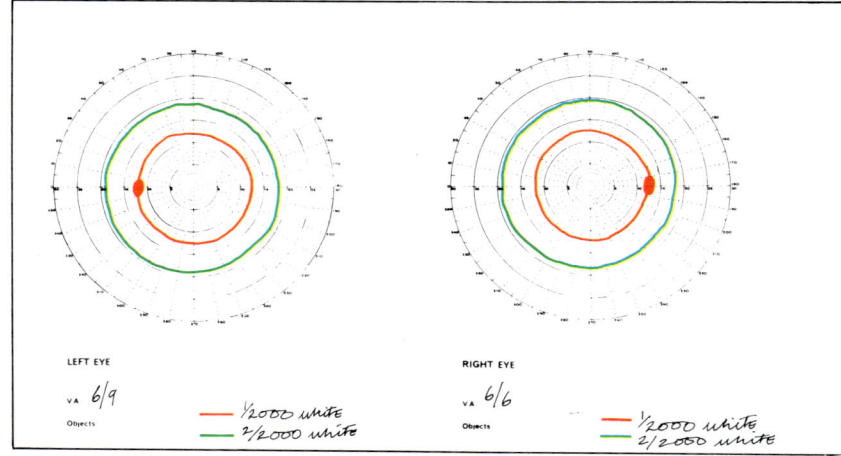

149 Tangent screen. The results are recorded on charts as the patient sees them. The usual targets are white discs of 1 or 2 mm in diameter, with the patient 2 m (2000 mm) away from the chart, which are recorded as 1w/2000 or 2w/2000 respectively. Larger targets may be required in patients with poor vision. A red target may be used. If the patient sits 2 m from the chart designed for the 1 m distance, the central 15° of field only are examined.

Goldmann-type perimeter

This examines the entire field of vision by bringing targets into view from around the patient. As with the tangent screen, the outer limits of the field are defined with kinetic perimetry (a moving target) and inner scotomas are sought by static perimetry.

Prior to use, both the stimulus and the background illumination should be calibrated so that when the test is repeated on different occasions, meaningful comparisons can be made. This should be done frequently, in a dark room.

Calibration

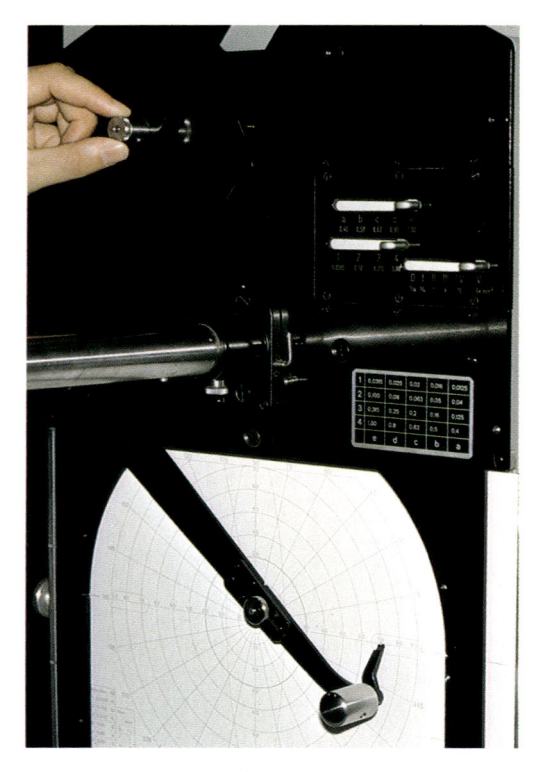

150

150 Stimulus calibration. The stimulus is calibrated first. The pointer is moved to 70° on the right and locked with the knob on the pointer arm as shown. This directs the stimulus at the photometer. All levers should be to the right i.e. on V-4e (brightest light).

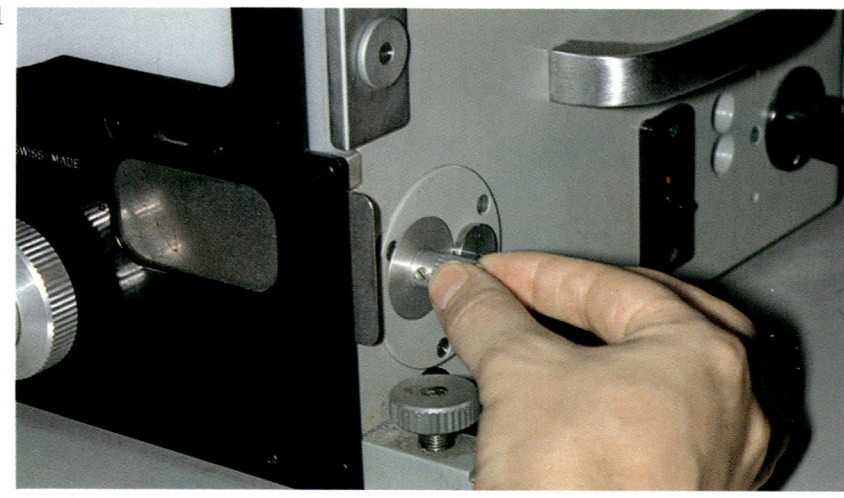

151 Stimulus calibration. The knob on the right side is turned so that the stimulus light is permanently on.

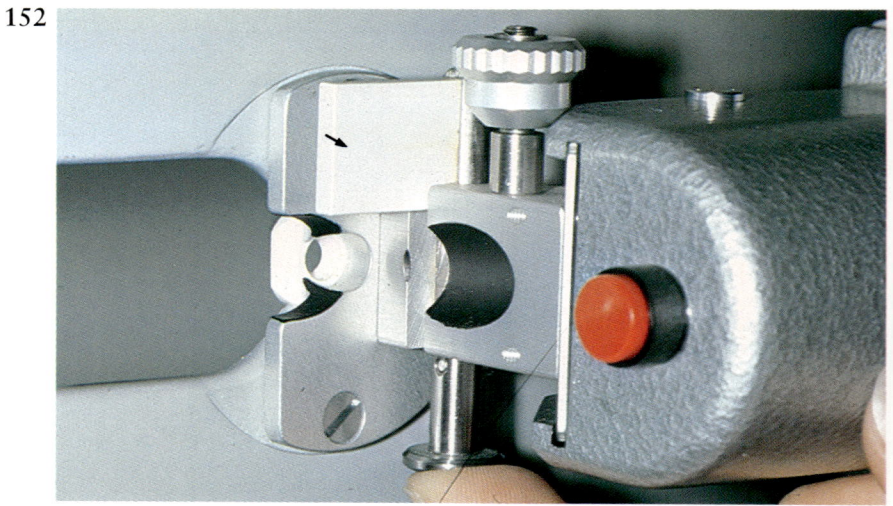

152 Stimulus calibration. The light meter is inserted at the left hand slot of the bowl and the photometer screen (arrow) raised.

153 Stimulus calibration. The stimulus rheostat, which is the knob further from the examiner on the left hand side of the instrument, is adjusted until the light meter reads 1,000 asb. (The scale is illuminated with a push button adjacent to it.) If it will not reach 1,000 asb, the stimulus may not be on or may be badly positioned, or the bulb may need replacing.

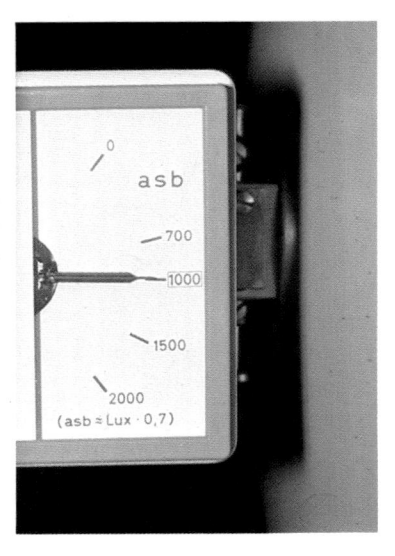

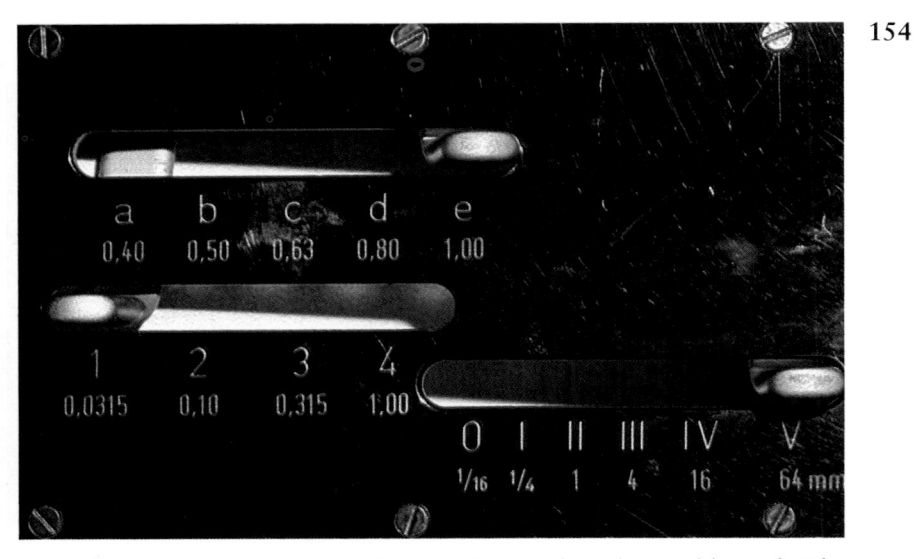

154 Background calibration. The background is then calibrated. The V-1e stimulus is used, which has an intensity of 32.5 asb, and the background illumination is adjusted to match this level.

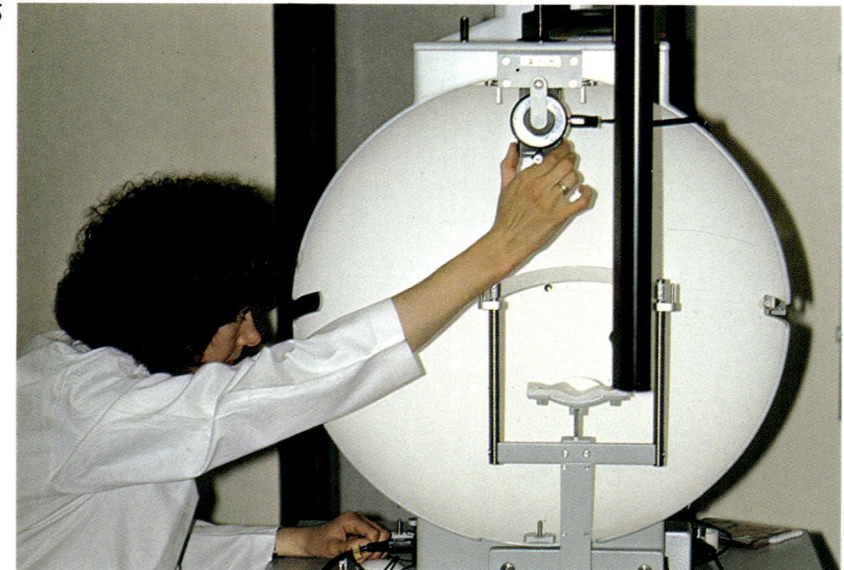

155 Background calibration. The photometer screen is lowered. The observer looks through the notch on the far side of the hemisphere at the photometer screen. The lampshade is adjusted with one hand.

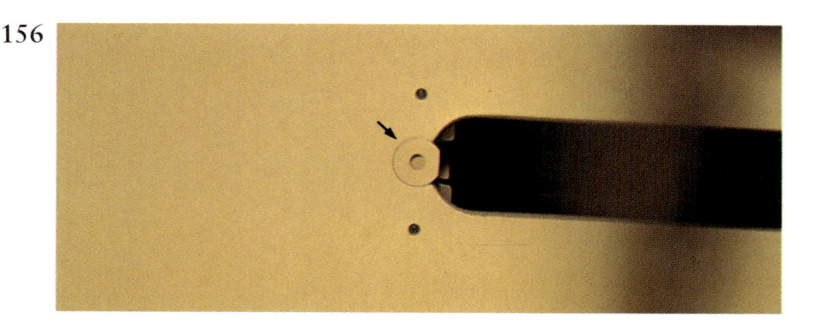

156 Background calibration. The ring that is seen (arrow) represents the background, and the centre of the ring is where the stimulus light falls, which has a known intensity. The shade is adjusted until the ring matches its centre. The background is then correctly calibrated, the photometer can be removed and the pointer handle unlocked.

Perimetry
After calibration, perimetry can begin. There are six sizes of target, 0-V (in Roman numerals), four original stimulus intensities in 0.5 log unit steps, 1-4, and five additional filter intensities in 0.1 log unit steps, a-e. Targets commonly used are:

Initially I-4e ('one four eee'), i.e. a 0.25 sq mm, 1,000 asb target; I-2e provided the above is seen, i.e. a 0.25 sq mm, 100 asb target; IV-4e if the smaller targets are not seen, i.e. a 16 sq mm 1,000 asb target.

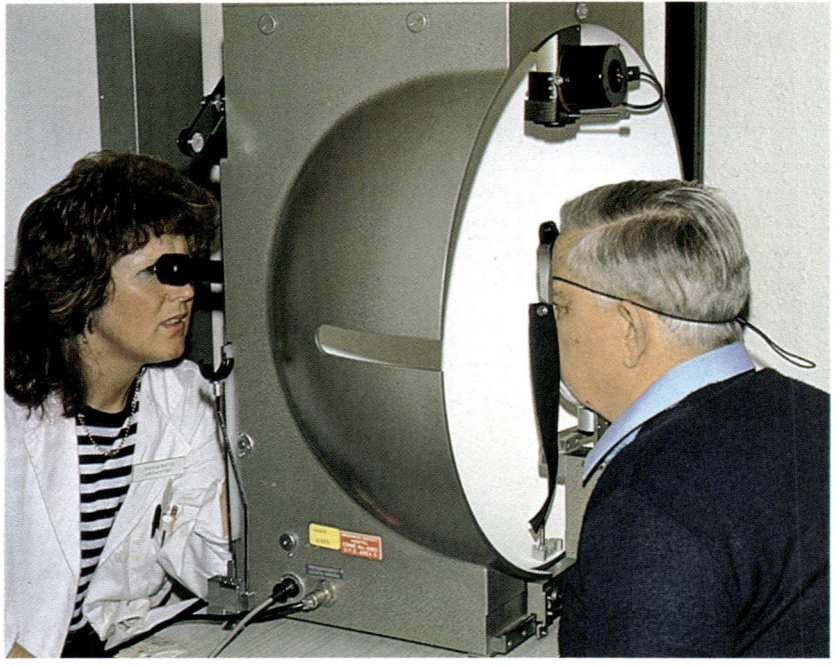

157 Goldmann-type perimetry. The patient is seated comfortably at the perimeter holding the indicator buzzer. One eye is occluded, the other eye centred by moving the chin rest, and the chart paper is inserted.

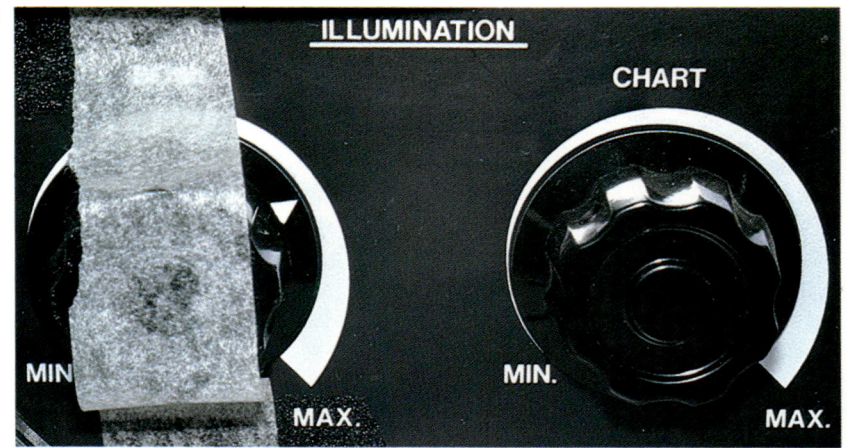

158 Goldmann-type perimetry. The chart illumination is controlled by the knob to the left of the instrument nearer the operator. This is easily confused with the rheostat for calibration; it is helpful to stick the latter down with tape once calibration is complete.

Peripheral isopters
The shutter controlling the stimulus on/off (**151**) should be set so that the stimulus is on when the shutter is depressed. The patient is asked to fix the central marker, and press the buzzer when he is aware of a light in his field of vision. The operator sets the stimulus size and intensity (e.g. to I-4e), then brings the pointer in from the extreme edge of the field at a slow even speed towards fixation. The patient's eye is simultaneously observed through the telescope to ascertain that fixation is indeed on the central marker. When the buzzer is pressed, a mark is made on the chart and the process repeated in another meridian. To move the stimulus arm from one side to the other it must be swung around the bottom of the chart.

Scotomas and blind spot

Once two peripheral isopters are plotted (usually I-4e and I-2e), the centre is examined for scotomas by placing the pointer in a likely area, then briefly depressing the shutter to illuminate the stimulus. The central 20° with an extension to 30° nasally is appropriate for most purposes; this is where early scotomas occur in glaucoma. The vertical meridian is explored in suspected chiasmal or post-chiasmal disease.

When a scotoma is found, it is demarcated by moving the target outwards from the blind area in several directions until the limits of the scotoma are defined. The blind spot is also mapped out in this manner. For the central 20° of field the patient will require his usual distance correction and a near add if he uses one for reading. Wide aperture lenses should be used. Aphakic eyes should be corrected with contact lenses.

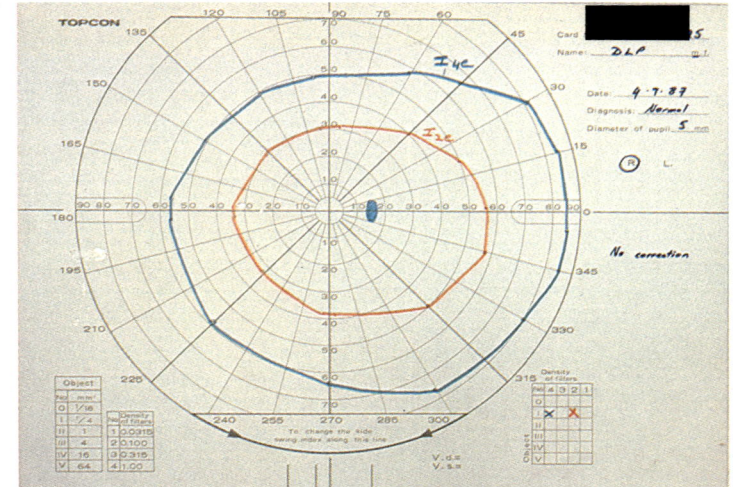

159 **Goldmann perimetry.** Normal field (right).

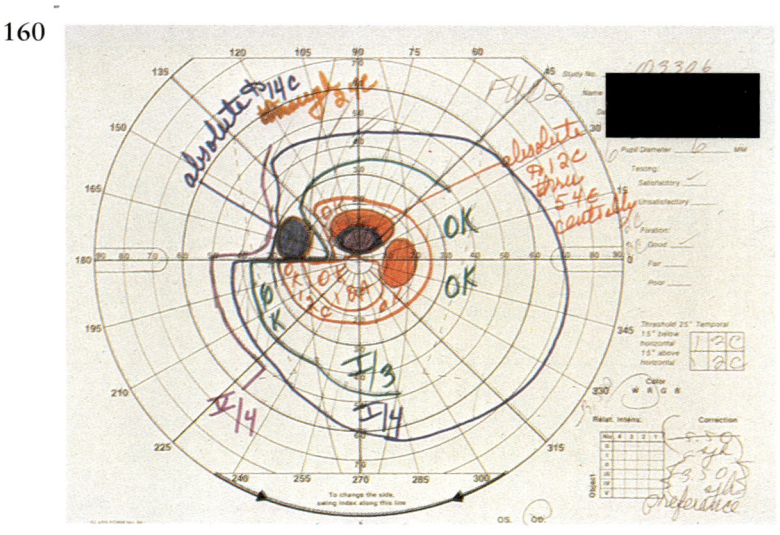

160 **Goldmann perimetry.** Abnormal field (right)—open angle glaucoma.

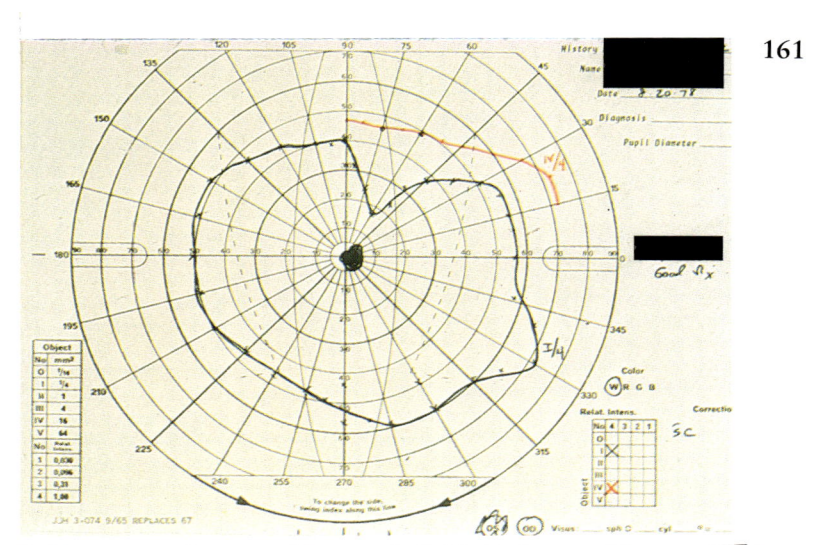

161 Goldmann perimetry. Abnormal field (right)—syndrome of the distal optic nerve (anterior chiasmal syndrome).

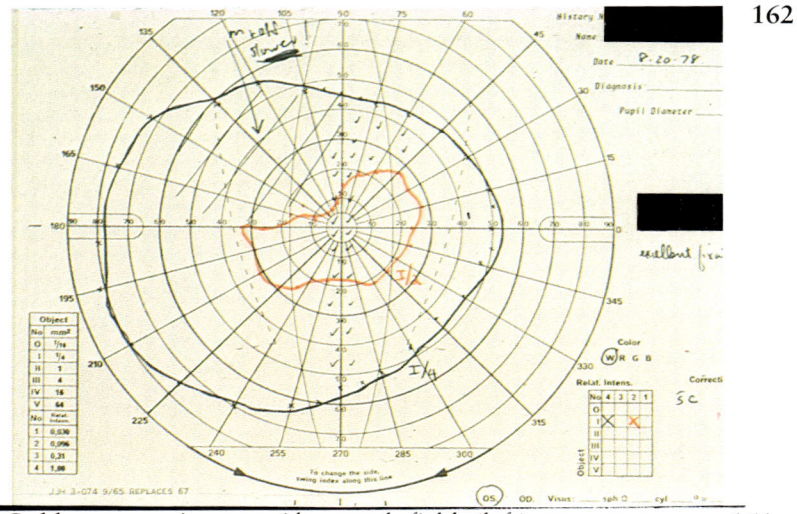

162 Goldmann perimetry. Abnormal field (left)—same case as **161** showing the junctional scotoma.

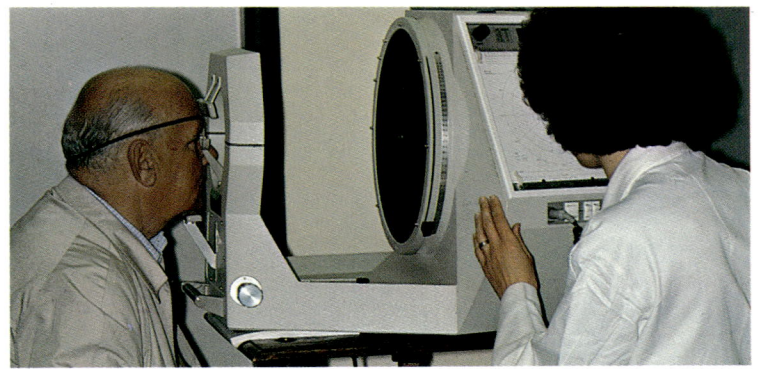

163 Friedmann analyser. The patient is seated and one eye is occluded. Wide aperture lenses are used to provide a correction as for the Goldmann-type perimeter.

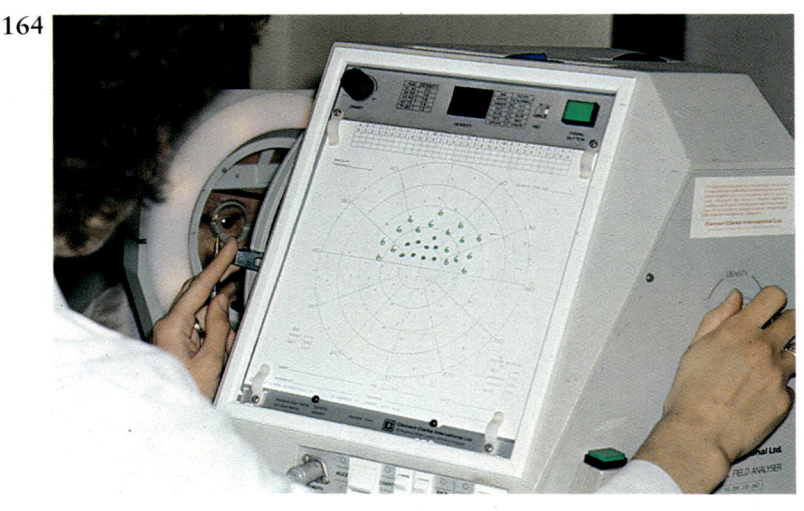

164 Friedmann analyser. The stimuli are presented by moving a lever (on the left) through numerous positions at a filter density (varied at right) appropriate for the patient's age or calibrated to be 0.4-0.6 log units above central threshold. Those stimuli that are missed are represented at a lesser filter density, i.e. a brighter stimulus. The filter setting required for visibility at each point is marked on the chart.

Friedmann analyser
This tests only the central 25° of field but is very sensitive, reproducible and easy to use without the interpretive effort necessary in the tangent screen or the Goldmann-type perimeter. A cluster of lights of variable location and intensity is presented briefly to the patient who simply states how many he sees. The size of the target is reduced nearer the centre of the field to compensate for increased retinal sensitivity. A few minutes dark adaptation should take place before the test. The equipment can also be used for dark adaptometry.

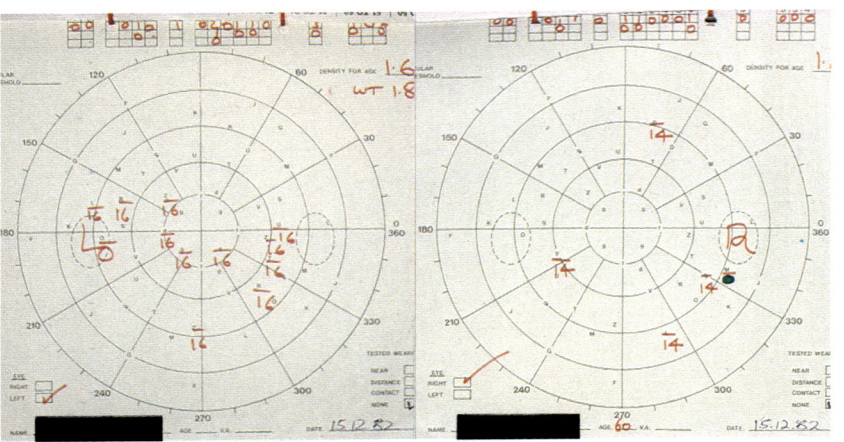

165 Friedmann analyser. The fields of a 60-year-old patient with raised intraocular pressure are shown.

An overall depression over time may be due to opacities in the media, most commonly increasing cataract, so the chart must be interpreted with the overall clinical picture in mind. Macular function can be tested by using the central aperture to ascertain the macular threshold. A macular grid examination can be performed using a red filter which may be of use in monitoring chloroquine therapy.

Automated perimetry

Automatic perimeters use static stimuli of fixed size, usually 4 sq mm (Goldmann size III) and commonly have a background illumination of 32 asb like the Goldmann perimeter. Three luminance strategies are possible in testing: threshold (which is probably too time-consuming for routine use); threshold-related supra-threshold (which is probably the most sensitive strategy); or supra-threshold (which is arbitrarily chosen but which may fail to detect early visual field loss). The automated system presents the stimuli at various preset locations and records whether the patient responds or not. If not, the stimulus is usually presented again at a greater intensity. Different programmes can be used, testing the field to a varying extent, e.g. the whole field or only the centre, or by varying the number of stimuli per unit area. A disadvantage of automation is that elderly patients may find the programmes too lengthy or inflexible and may therefore perform less well.

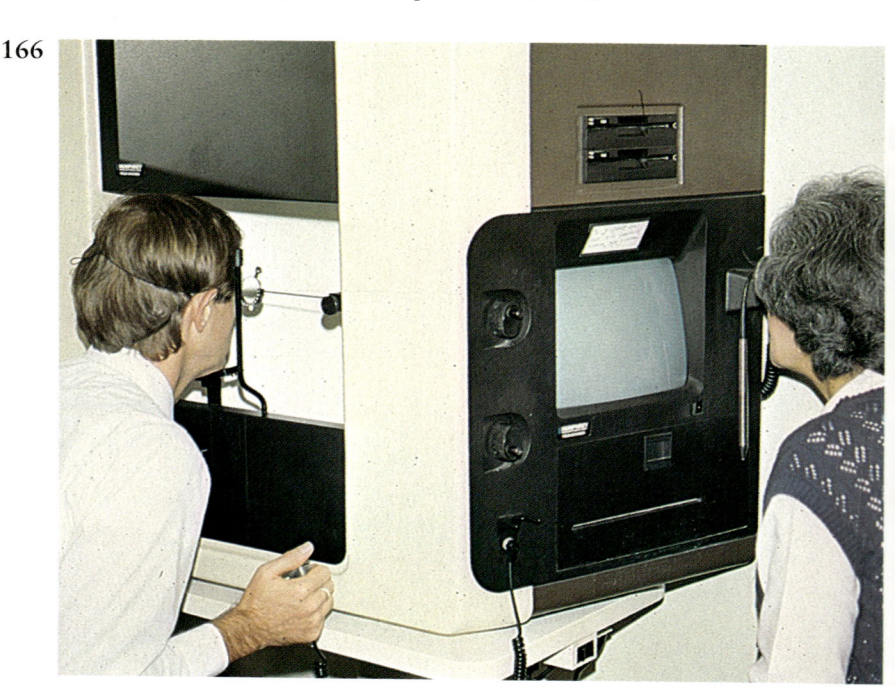

166 Automated perimeter. The Humphrey instrument is shown.

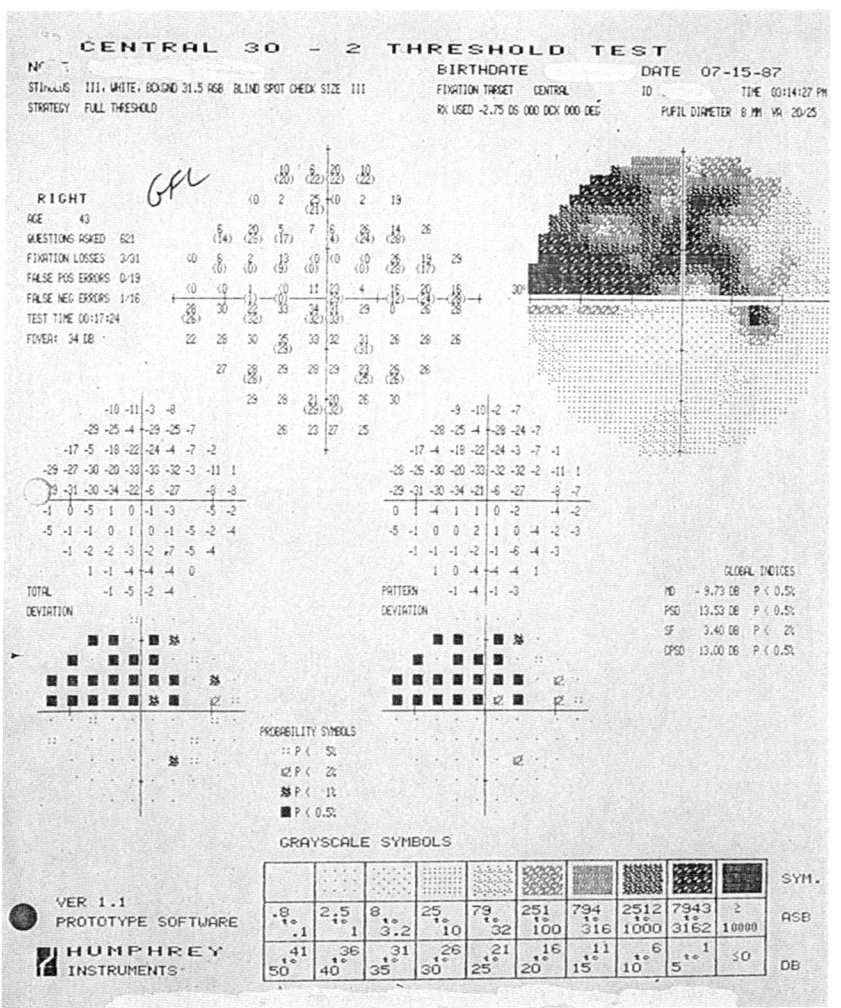

167 Automated perimeter. Abnormal field—open angle glaucoma. The results may be printed numerically, or as a greyscale giving the pattern of the field at a glance.

Gonioscopy

Gonioscopy is performed to examine the angle in all patients with raised intra-ocular pressure, and in some other instances, e.g. melanoma of the iris. Field tests should be done prior to gonioscopy, and dilatation if planned deferred until afterwards.

The Goldmann gonioscopy lens is illustrated here. Its application to the cornea permits a view of the angle opposite the mirror. The central portion of the lens provides a view of the posterior pole, which is ideal for examining the disc at the same time as the angle if pupil size permits.

One alternative lens is the Koeppe lens in which the angle is viewed directly rather than through a mirror. Another alternative is the Zeiss four-mirror lens which can artificially open a closed angle with pressure, to demonstrate reversible or irreversible closure.

The procedure is explained to the patient and local anaesthetic applied.

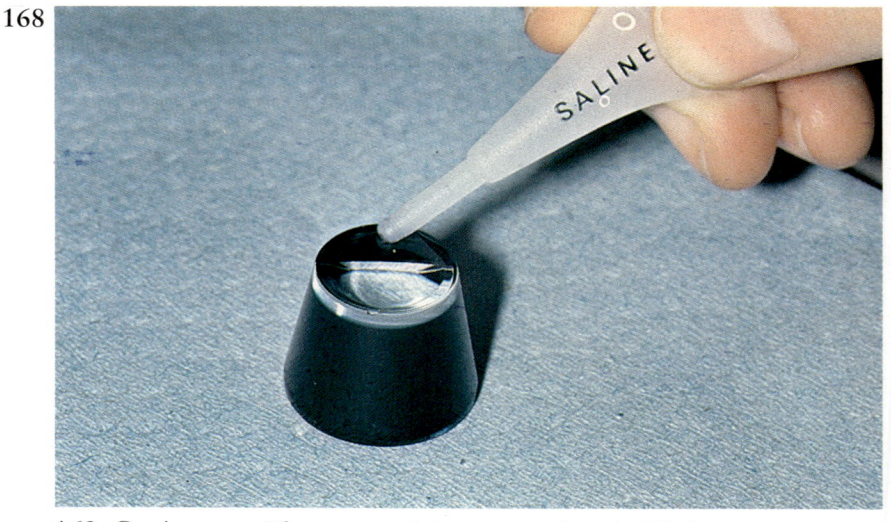

168 Gonioscopy. The centre of the contact lens is filled with saline or 2 per cent methyl cellulose. Saline disturbs the epithelium less, permitting a clearer subsequent view of the fundus but methyl cellulose is more viscous and easier for the inexperienced user.

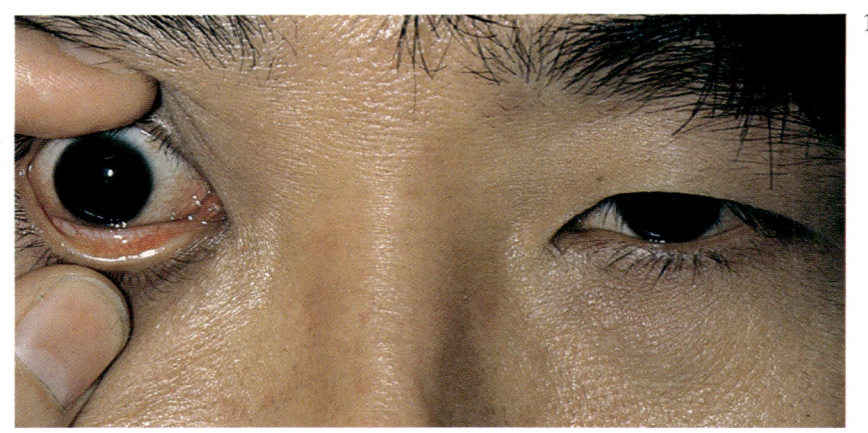

169 Gonioscopy. The patient is positioned at the slit-lamp. He is asked to gently close his eyes. The index finger is firmly placed on the upper lid margin. The patient is then asked to open his eyes and the lid is raised with the index finger. Mild upward pressure over the tarsal plate will prevent the patient closing his eye while the lens is being inserted. The thumb holds the weaker lower lid open.

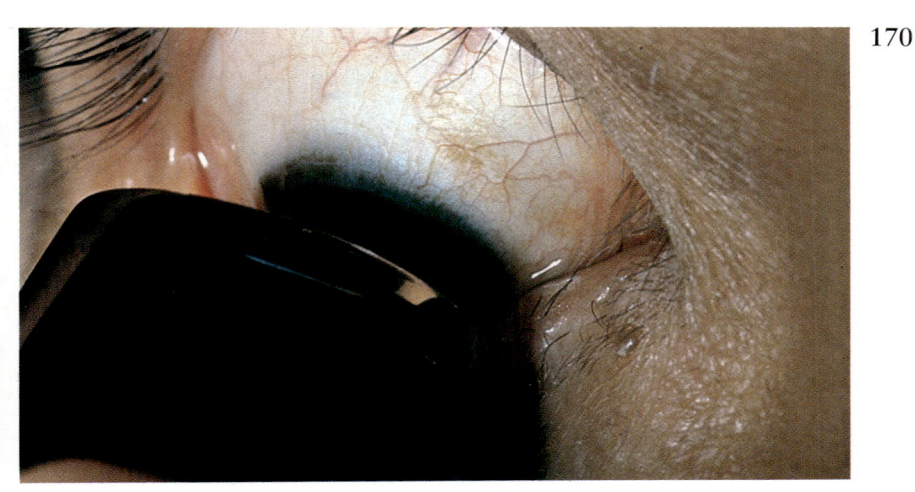

170 Gonioscopy. The patient is asked to look down and the lower edge of the gonioscopy lens is inserted into the lower fornix.

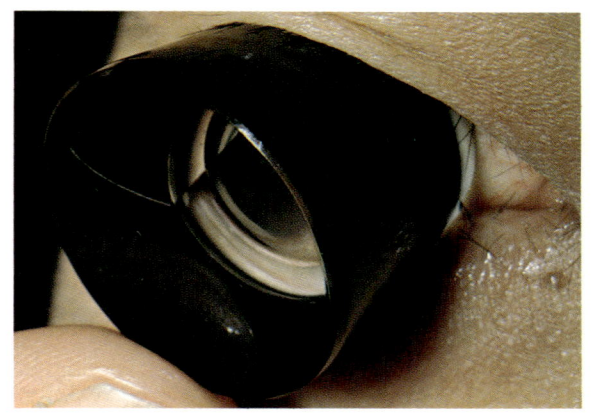

171 Gonioscopy. The whole lens is then rocked onto the cornea. If a bubble has appeared between the lens and the eye, the process is repeated making sure the patient looks well down so the fluid does not dribble out.

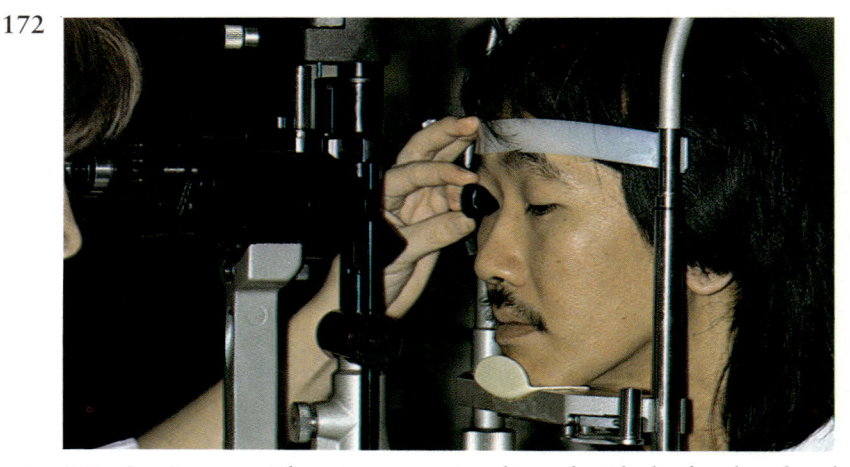

172 Gonioscopy. The microscope is adjusted with the free hand to focus upon the reflection of the angle in the mirror. The magnification is increased. The angle that is seen is located exactly opposite the mirror. The lens is rotated on the eye and the slit beam aimed perpendicular to the angle. The beam may be narrowed and the lens tilted to reduce reflections. A view into a narrow angle is provided by asking the patient to look in the direction of the mirror. If the angle structures are visible, the angle is open.

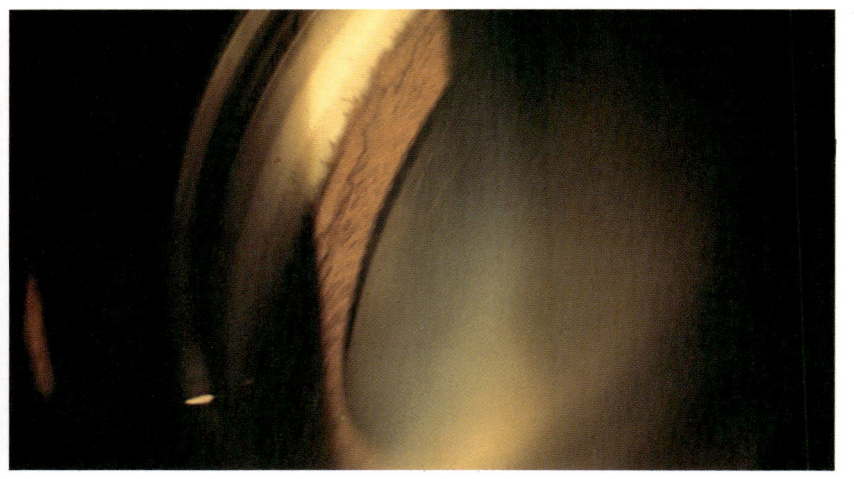

173 Gonioscopy. An open angle.

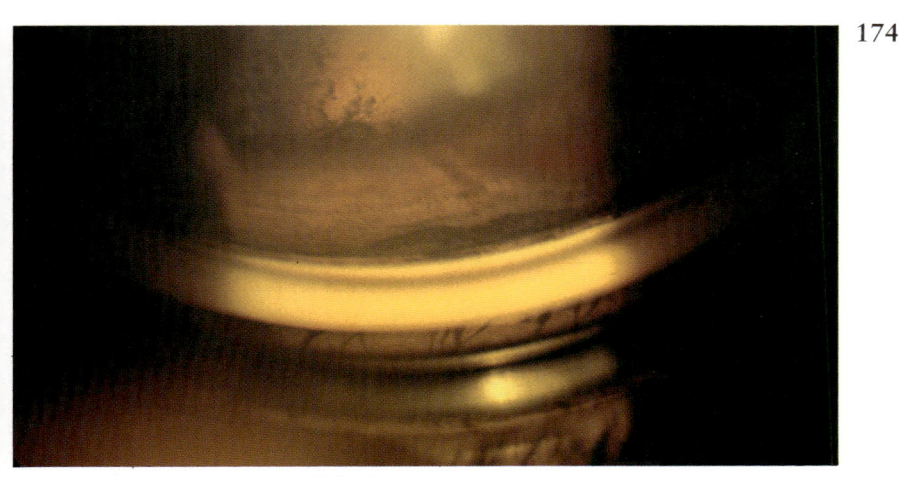

174 Gonioscopy. An iris dialysis.

All four quadrants should be examined in both eyes and the results recorded immediately before they are confused. Grading systems may be used, but a simple alternative is to describe how much of the angle is seen in each quadrant; e.g. supero-nasal quadrant: trabecular meshwork visible.

10 Tests for posterior segment diagnosis

Amsler chart

Where a macular (or optic nerve) lesion is suspected it is customary to use the Amsler chart to detect a central field abnormality. This is done before dilatation for fundus examination.

The chart is viewed at reading distance (30 cm). The patient wears a near correction if usual and one eye is occluded. He is asked if he sees the central dot on the page, and to describe whether any parts of the surrounding grid are distorted or blurred in any way. This will detect abnormalities in the central 10° of field. If the dot is not seen, a chart marked with a large cross is used so that the patient knows where it should be.

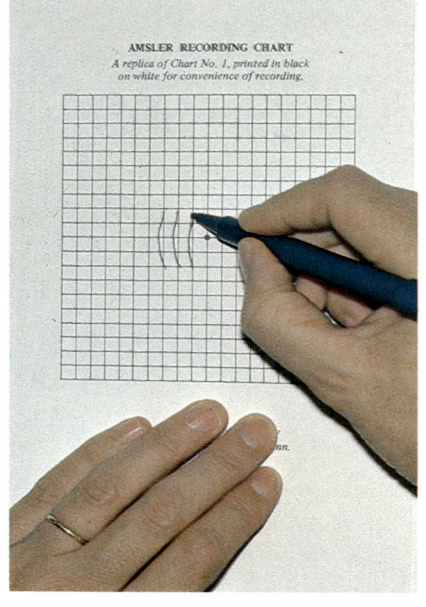

175 Amsler chart. The patient can mark off abnormal areas with a pen, while still looking at the central dot. The standard charts are white lines on a black background but the tear-off recording charts of black lines on a white background as illustrated are suitable for this purpose.

Direct ophthalmoscopy

The direct ophthalmoscope's principal assets are the magnification it provides (about × 15) and its ease of use. It is used to examine the disc and vessels for detail, e.g. disc swelling, new vessels in diabetics. The pupil does not need to be dilated to see the disc with the direct ophthalmoscope but dilatation is necessary to view the macula. A red-free (green) filter is an asset particularly in viewing the nerve fibre layer.

176 Direct ophthalmoscopy. The larger strength lenses (1) are set to 0. The smaller strength lenses in the instrument (2) are set to the plus side e.g. + 10D. This will allow the observer to focus on anterior segment structures initially.

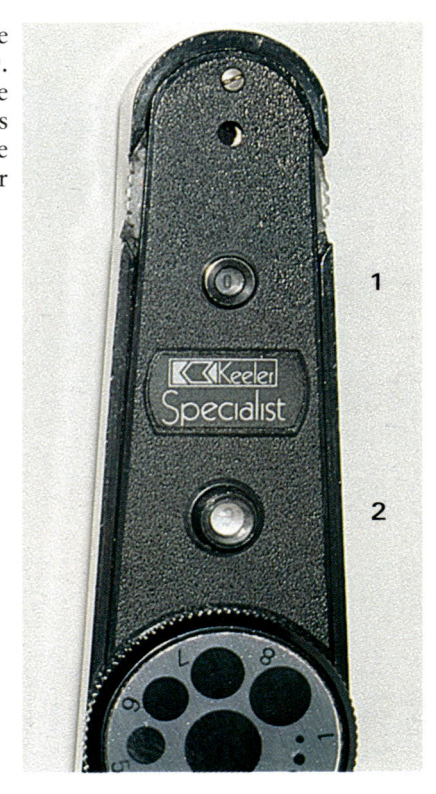

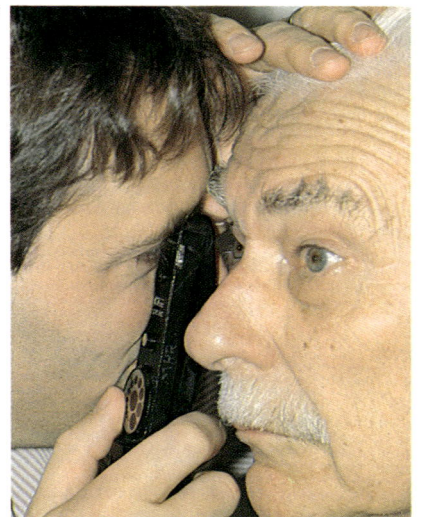

177 Direct ophthalmoscopy. If the right eye is to be examined the observer uses his right eye and the left eye for the left. The observer approaches the eye, shifting the lenses from +10 down towards 0. The cornea and lens will come into focus and then the fundus. With an emmetropic patient and examiner the added lens strength will be 0. The closer the examiner is to the patient the larger will be his field of view, therefore he should approach very near as shown. In high ametropia or astigmatism the fundus may be seen best through the patient's own glasses.

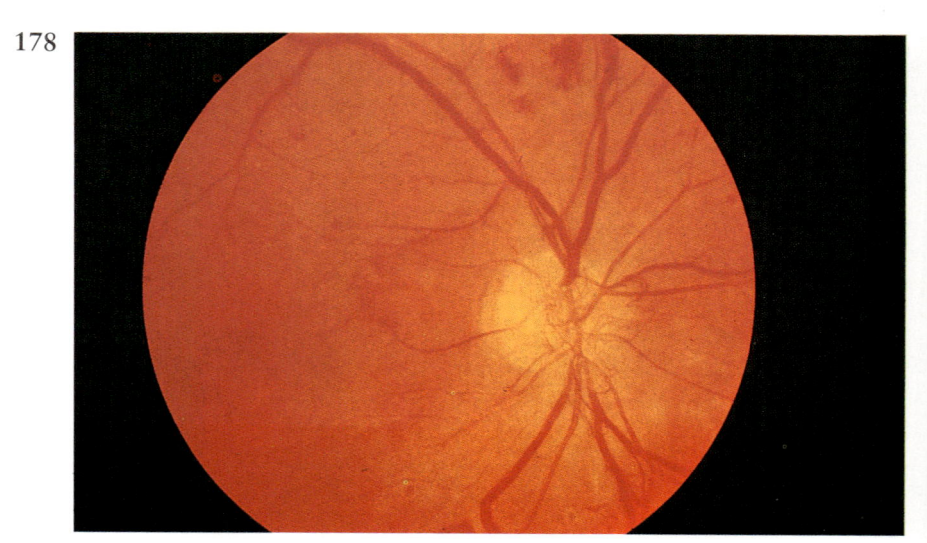

178 Fundal appearance. Disc pathology such as the diabetic neovascularization illustrated is examined with the direct ophthalmoscope.

Indirect ophthalmoscopy

The main advantage of the indirect ophthalmoscope is its wide field of view compared to the direct, permitting examination of the retinal periphery. It provides considerably less magnification, only about 3 × if a 20 dioptre lens is used (depending on the viewing distance and the patient's refraction). The view is stereoscopic. It should be used prior to diagnostic contact lens insertion so that a disturbed corneal epithelium does not obscure the view.

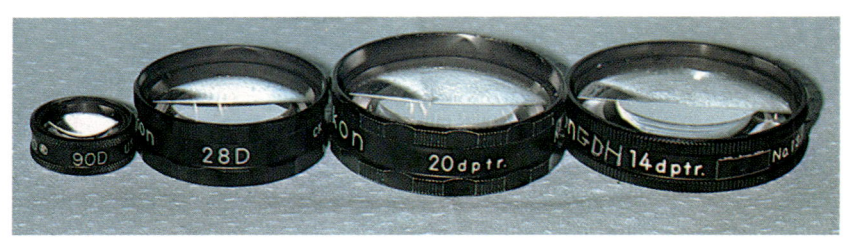

179 Lenses. The 20 dioptre lens is used most of the time. The 28 dioptre lens is helpful if the pupil will not dilate but provides less magnification. The 14 dioptre lens provides more magnification but positioning is more critical. (The 90 dioptre lens is used with the slit-lamp.) The lenses are held with the white rim facing the patient or the more curved surface away from the patient, and must be clean.

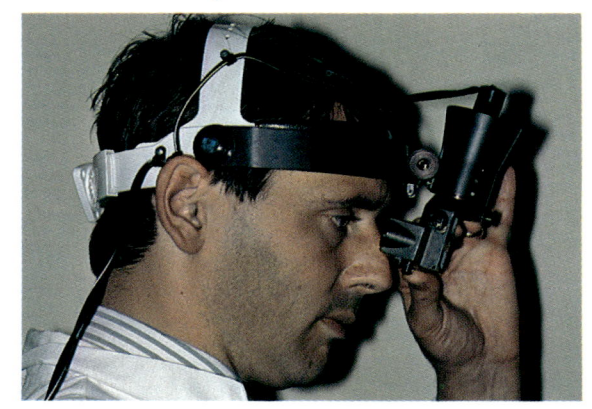

180 Indirect ophthalmoscopy. The headband is placed on the examiner's head and adjusted to fit comfortably. The component consisting of the light, the two eyepieces and the reflecting mirror, is lowered and the interpupillary distance adjusted so that the examiner has a clear binocular, symmetrical view of his thumb at arm's length through the eyepieces.

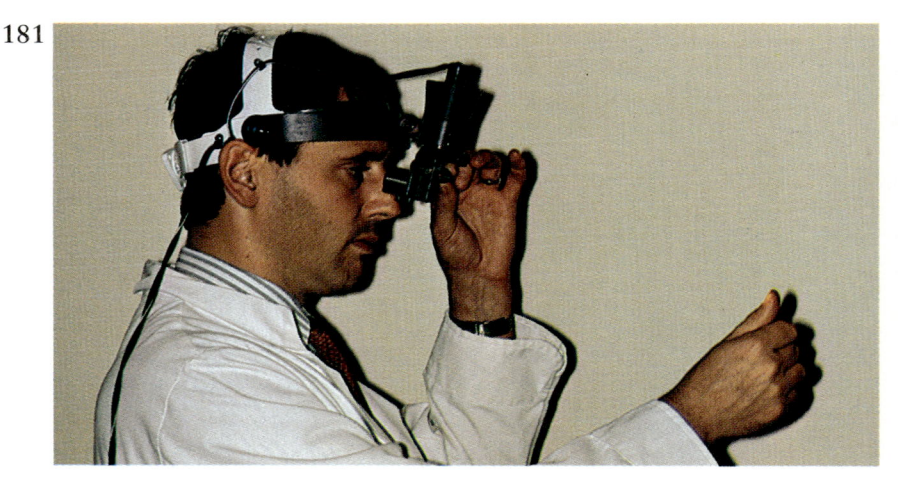

181 Indirect ophthalmoscopy. Still holding his thumb out at arm's length before him, the examiner adjusts the mirror to direct the light onto his thumb.

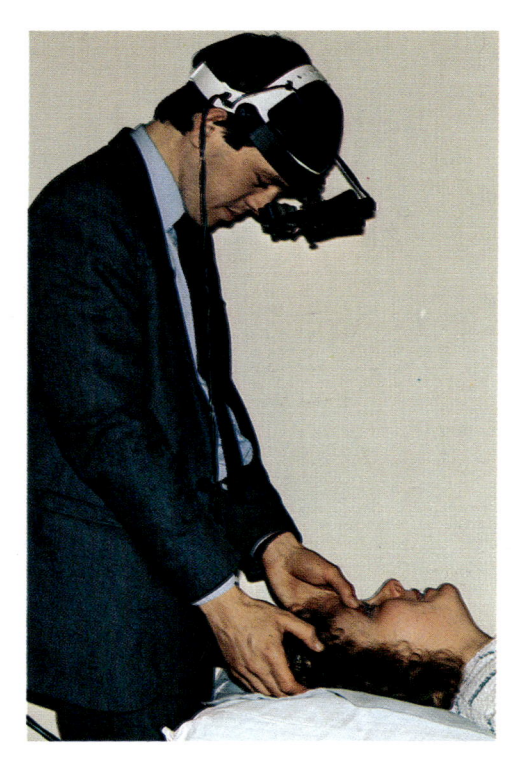

182 Indirect ophthalmoscopy. The patient's pupils are dilated and he lies on a couch. The examiner stands straight at the patient's head and instructs him to look at the ceiling above. The lids are held apart and the examiner bends his head forward so that the light from the indirect ophthalmoscope shines vertically down at the pupil. A red reflex should be seen. If examining the seated patient, the examiner sits opposite the patient at the same level, maintaining the same alignment as for a patient lying down.

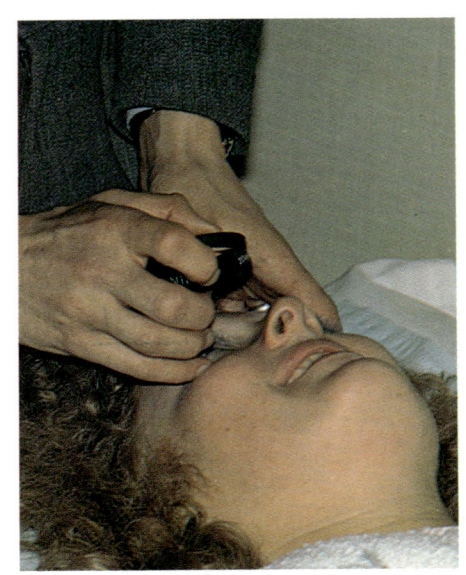

183 Indirect ophthalmoscopy. The lens is then interposed between the eye and the light source, approximately at right angles to the light beam. The examiner's hand rests lightly on the patient's face to control the lens movement. If the lens is held near the eye the pupil is seen, and on raising the lens the pupil margins will disappear and the whole fundus will appear. Small variations in height are significant.

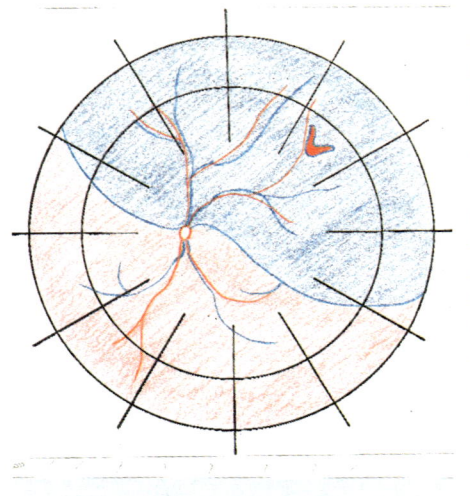

184 Retinal drawing. The disc, macula and vessels should be identified. The image is seen to be inverted. This is best appreciated by drawing exactly what is seen in the lens, while standing at the head of the patient, with an inverted chart relative to the patient; the macula appears to be on the nasal side. The drawing represents what is seen in the direct ophthalmoscope with the examiner face to face with the patient.

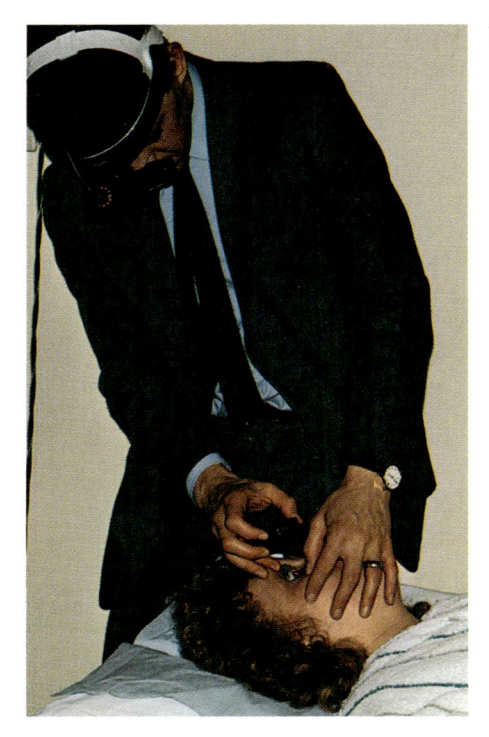

185 Peripheral retinal examination. The periphery is examined by asking the patient to look in the required direction. The examiner bends away from the patient's direction of gaze, so angling the light beam to the area to be viewed. The lens is still held approximately at right angles to the beam. Orientation may be difficult; the position of the eye is the determining factor, i.e. if the patient is looking inferotemporally, the inferotemporal retina is that being examined, however confusing the image may appear. The peripheral features are also added to the drawing.

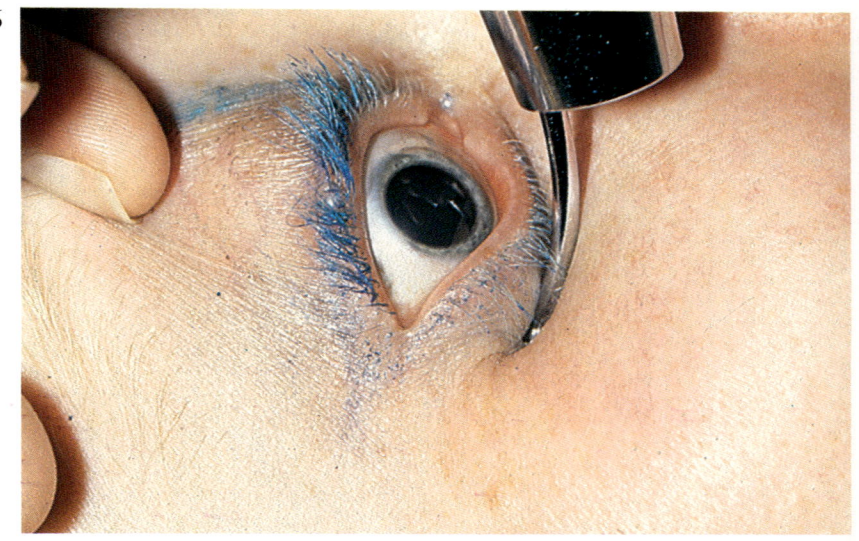

186 Scleral depression. This is necessary to see the ora serrata and pars plana. The depressor is gently placed on the lid, which it also retracts. The observer views the retinal periphery while he glides the tip backwards on the globe, seeing the indented area as a paler elevation. This procedure should not be painful and does not require an anaesthetic. The medial canthus cannot be indented but this area can be seen when the eye is slightly elevated or depressed.

Use of the slit-lamp with accessory lenses

The lenses are contact or non-contact, and positive or negative. A dim beam and low magnification are used until the desired area is seen and the beam parameters are then adjusted.

Non-contact lenses

Hruby lens
This is a -58.6 dioptre lens which offers a stereoscopic view of the posterior pole through a dilated pupil, providing a 1:1 magnification. Up to 30° vertically and 60° laterally can be seen.

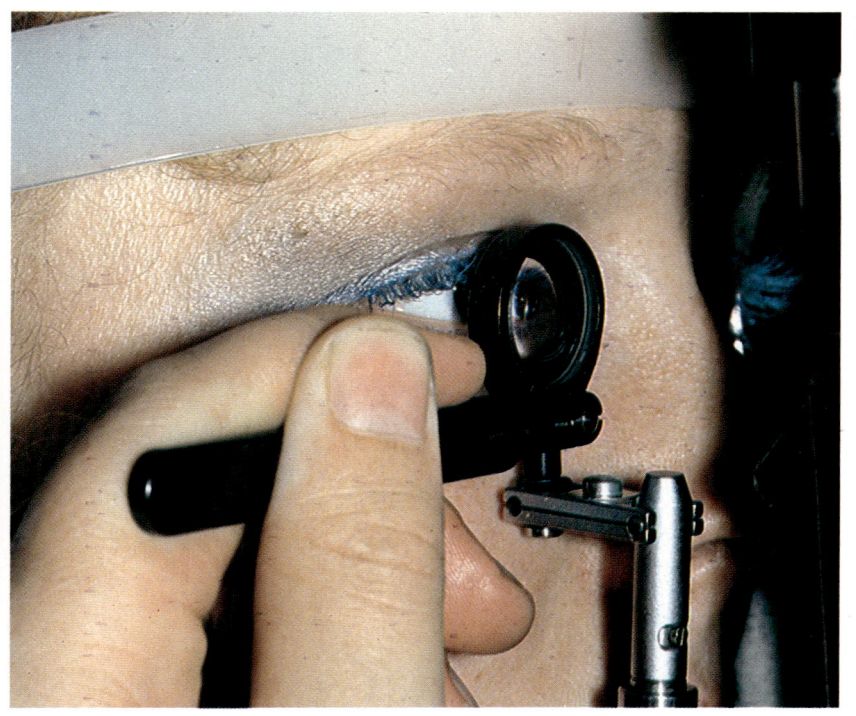

187 Hruby lens. The patient watches the fixation light with the other eye, beginning in the primary position. The clean Hruby lens is inserted into its support, with the flatter lens surface facing the observer.

The slit beam is aligned nearly axially. Using the attached strut, the lens is moved as close to the eye as possible without actually touching it, keeping it parallel to the observation path and centred on the eye. The examiner moves the microscope towards the patient until the fundus comes into focus and the posterior pole is surveyed. To obtain a more lateral view, the patient looks slightly to one side, the slit-lamp is swung a little to the other side and the Hruby is rotated to remain approximately perpendicular to the observation path.

A bright narrow beam with high magnification is used for perception of depth, especially for cystoid macular oedema or macular detachment where separation of the layers is seen.

+90 dioptre lens
As with the indirect ophthalmoscope, a real inverted image is produced by the positive lens. This is observed with the slit-lamp microscope. If used with a dilated pupil the periphery can be examined. It can be used with an undilated pupil, when only the disc and immediate surrounding area can be seen.

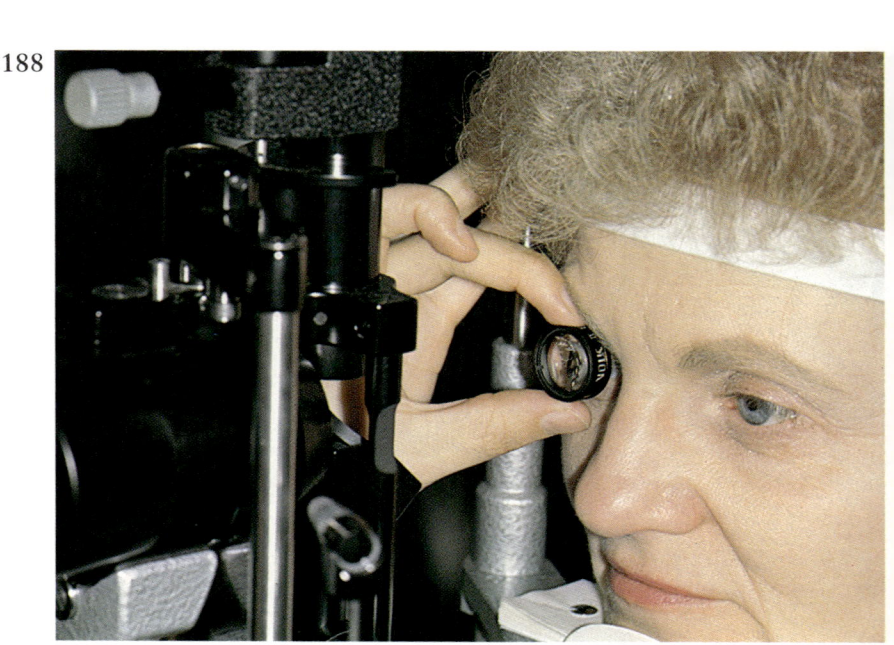

188

188 +90 lens. The beam is aligned axially and directed at the pupil centre. Looking through the eyepieces, the examiner focusses on the cornea. The +90 dioptre lens is then positioned just under 1 cm in front of the patient's cornea. The slit-lamp is drawn back by 1 in, using the joystick. This should produce a sharp retinal image. If it does not, the alignment must be checked again. Scanning is performed by moving the slit-lamp up and down, keeping the lens in place.

To examine the periphery, the patient is asked to gaze in the appropriate direction, the slit-lamp beam is realigned with the pupil, and the above steps repeated. Reflections may be reduced by tilting the +90 lens, or displacing the illuminating beam from the axis, or tilting the beam vertically, but all these variations must only be slight.

Diagnostic contact lenses

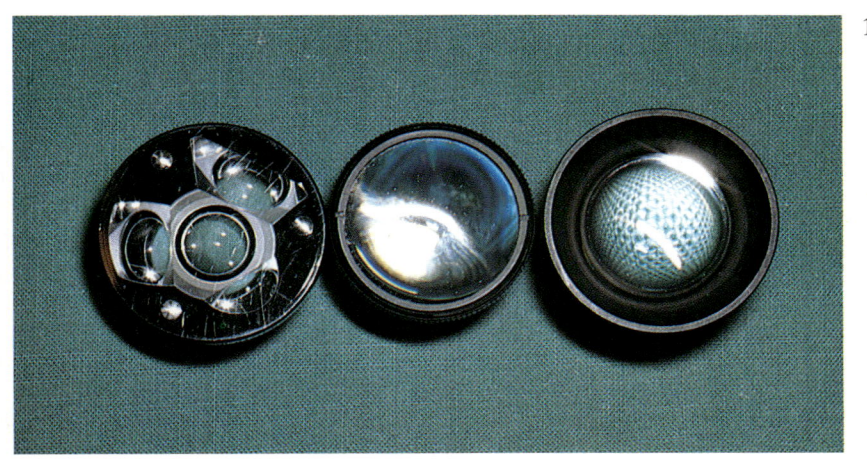

189 Diagnostic contact lenses. The Goldmann 3-mirror and two types of panfunduscope.

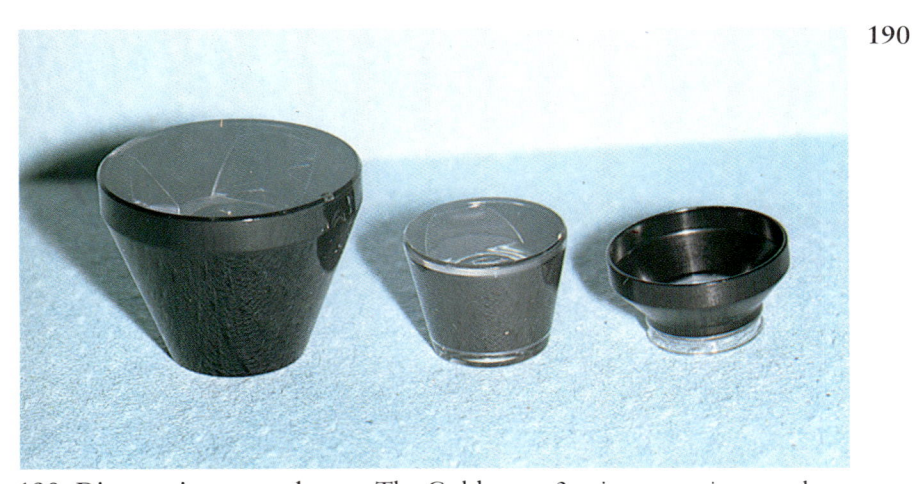

190 Diagnostic contact lenses. The Goldmann 3-mirror, gonioscopy lens and fundus contact lens.

Goldmann 3-mirror lens
This is a diagnostic contact lens with three mirrors of varying size and orientation (59°, 67° and 73°). The larger the mirror, the more angled towards the posterior pole. The smallest semicircular mirror corresponds to the gonioscope lens mirror. The central portion of the lens provides a direct magnified view of the posterior pole (not a reflected view). The 3-mirror lens is used to confirm retinal tears seen with the indirect ophthalmoscope, to seek further tears prior to surgery and to examine other peripheral retinal pathology. It is also used for laser therapy. It should not be used on the day retinal surgery is planned as its application may reduce corneal transparency.

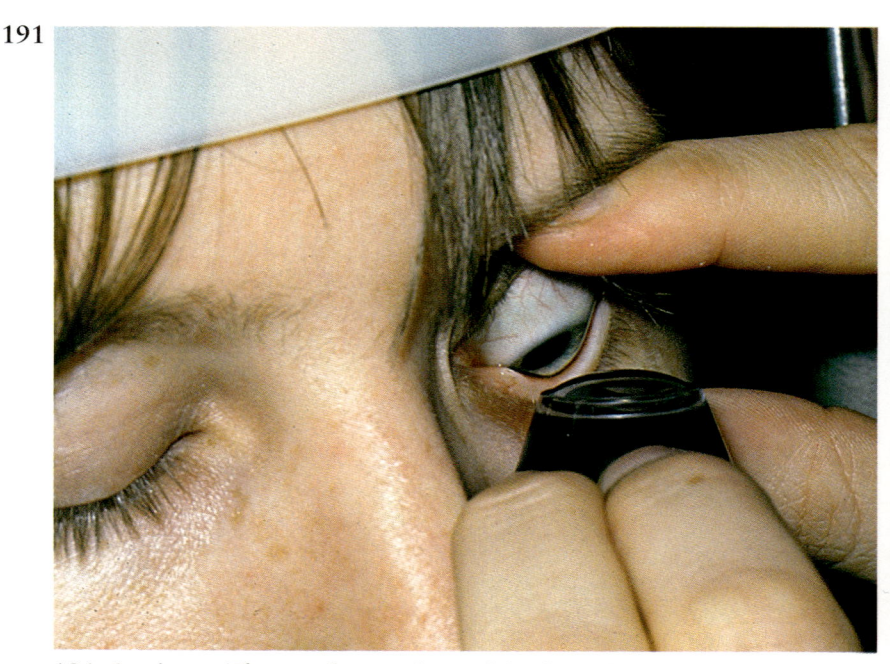

191 3-mirror. The pupil must be widely dilated. Topical anaesthetic is instilled into the eye and the patient seated at the slit-lamp. Saline or a 2 per cent methyl cellulose solution is used to fill the corneal surface of the lens. The upper lid is firmly controlled with the index finger on the tarsal plate and the lower lid with the thumb. The patient looks down, and the lip of the lens is gently inserted into the lower fornix.

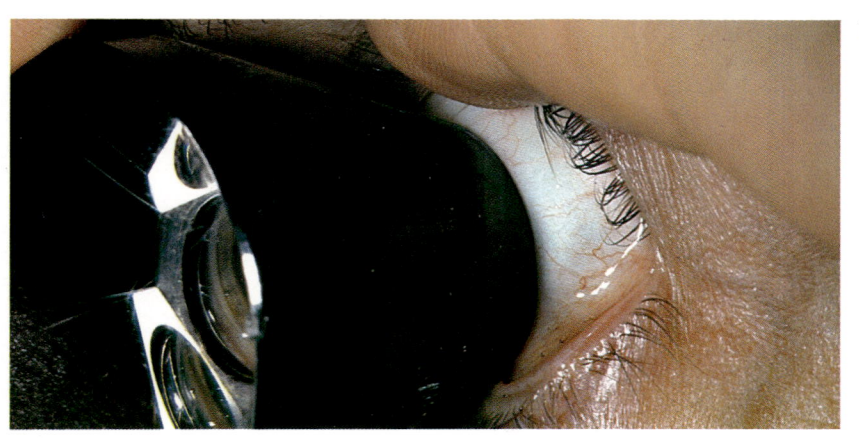

192 3-mirror. The whole lens is then tilted on to the cornea. If the upper lid is not properly controlled the lens will end up against the closed lid.

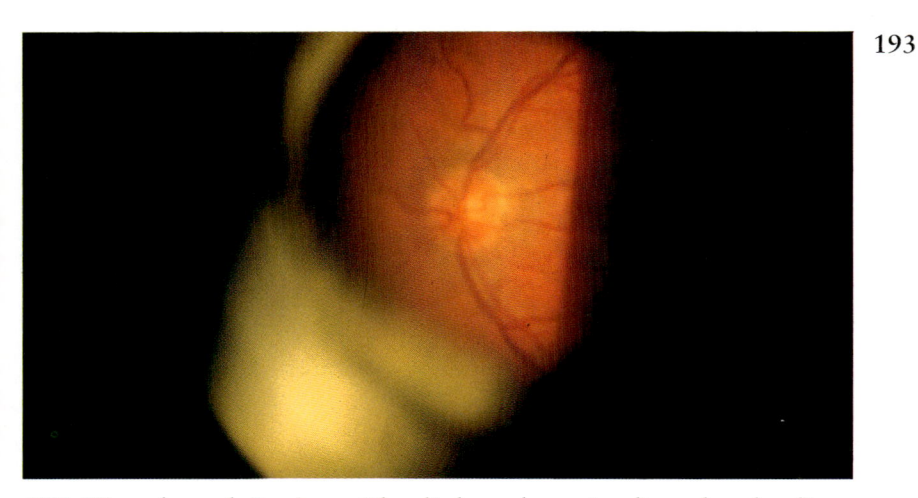

193 View through 3-mirror. The slit-lamp beam is adjusted under direct vision and the examiner then looks through the eyepieces to focus. A mirror image of the retina opposite, or the posterior pole as illustrated will be seen. The slit-beam can be turned obliquely or horizontally and tilted to facilitate viewing. The lens is removed by pressing gently on the lid to deform the globe beside the lens.

Fundus contact lens
The fundus contact lens is similar to the central portion of the Goldmann 3-mirror but is thinner and more manoeuvrable. It provides a view of 30° all around. In astigmatic patients and high myopes the fundus contact lens may provide a clearer image than the Hruby lens.

Panfunduscope
This is a positive contact lens which provides a view from one equator to another but with less magnification.

Ophthalmodynamometry

The pressure in the ophthalmic artery is related to the systemic blood pressure, the intravascular resistance and the intra-ocular pressure. A reduced ophthalmic artery pressure in one eye compared with the other suggests narrowing of the common carotid or the origin of the internal carotid on that side.

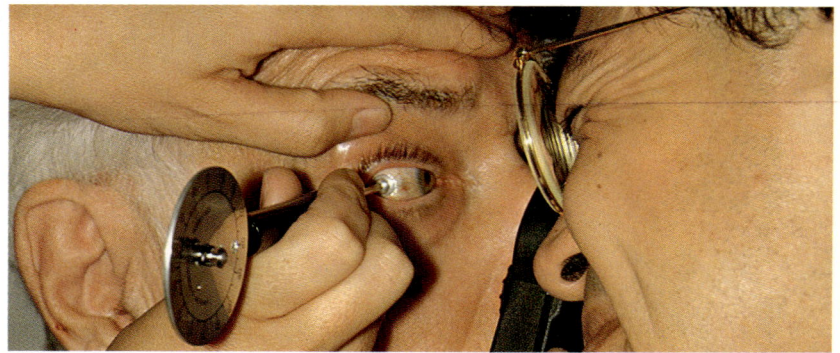

194 Ophthalmodynamometry. A local anaesthetic is applied. The examiner observes the central retinal artery through a direct or indirect ophthalmoscope. The clean ophthalmodynamometer is applied to the sclera and the pressure on the globe increased. When the central retinal artery begins to pulsate the intra-ocular pressure just exceeds the diastolic pressure in the ophthalmic artery and the scale is read. The pressure is elevated further until pulsations cease and the scale read again at the systolic pressure in the artery, then the instrument is removed. The procedure should be brief to avoid prolonged retinal ischaemia.

Ultrasonography

High frequency sound waves are differentially reflected from tissues and commonly displayed in a two-dimensional mode (B-mode) for diagnostic purposes, though a one-dimensional mode (A-mode) is used for biometry (Chapter 12).

The most routine diagnostic use of this procedure is to determine whether posterior segment pathology exists when the media are opaque. It is also of assistance in detecting intra-ocular foreign bodies subsequent to injury and elucidating the nature of intra-ocular or orbital masses, though with the advent of high definition CT scans it is used less in the orbit.

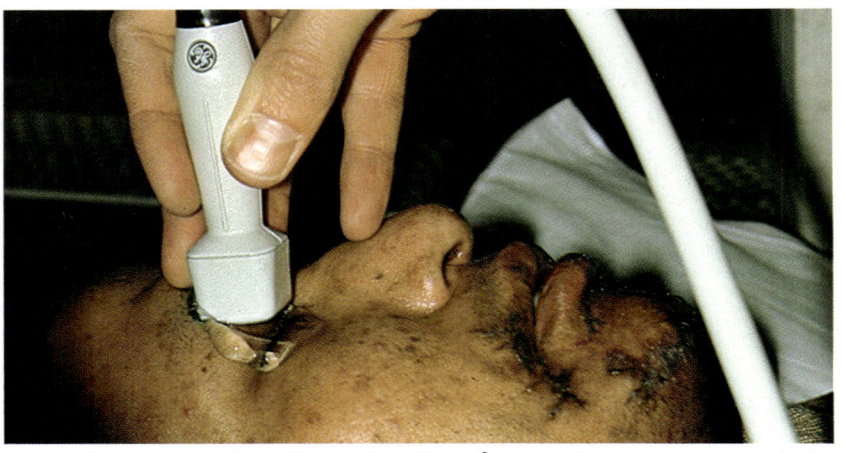

195 Ultrasonography. The patient lies on a couch with eyes closed. An aqueous gel is applied to the upper lid to improve contact. (Alternatively, a saline-bath coupling is available.) A hand-held transducer is placed either vertically or horizontally on the gel on the lid and an image appears on the screen. The globe is scanned with the transducer to identify the optic nerve and other structures.

The patient is asked to move his eyes to reveal the dynamic nature of intra-ocular shadows, e.g. a vitreous haemorrhage will move freely whereas a retinal detachment will not. A camera attachment is usually present to record the findings on polaroid film. The following illustrations are transverse, linear, saline-bath coupled B-scan sections.

196 Ultrasonography. Posterior vitreous detachment outlined by intragel haemorrhage (arrow).

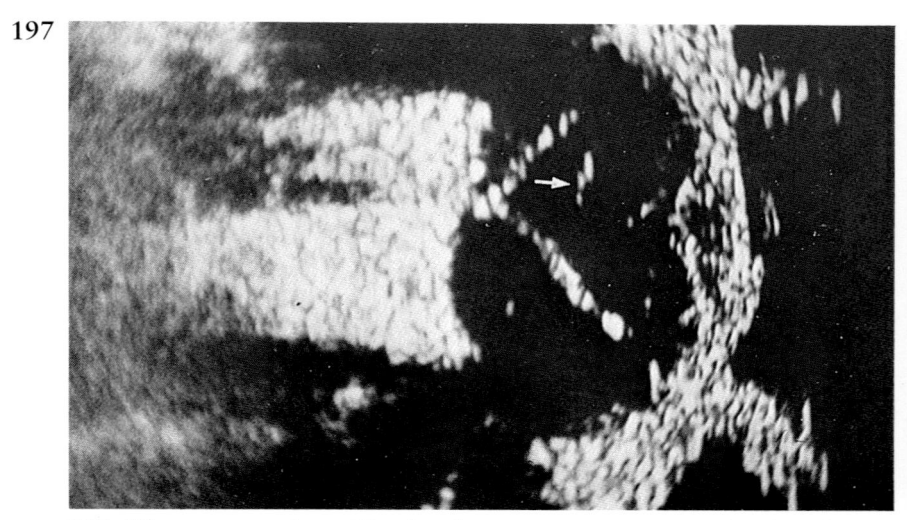

197 Ultrasonography. Total rhegmatogenous retinal detachment (V-shape); posterior vitreous detachment (arrow); cataractous lens.

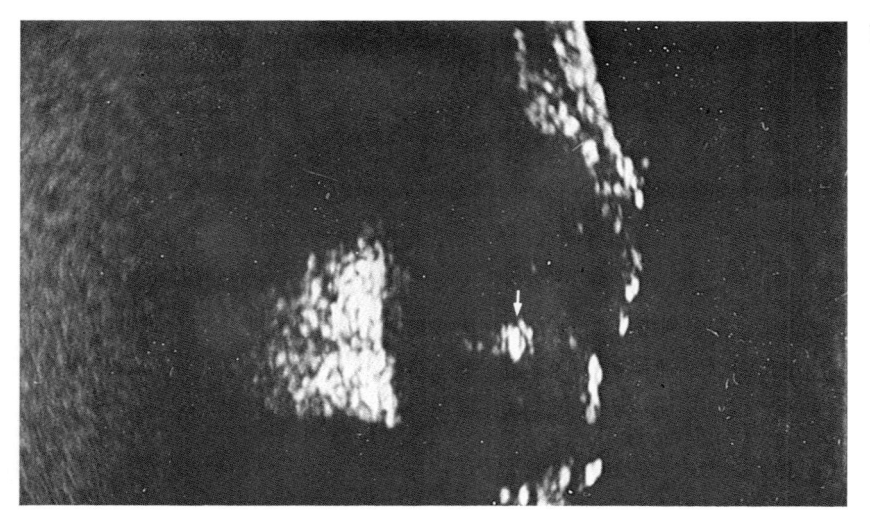

198 Ultrasonography. Foreign body in vitreous producing attenuation of sound beam (arrow).

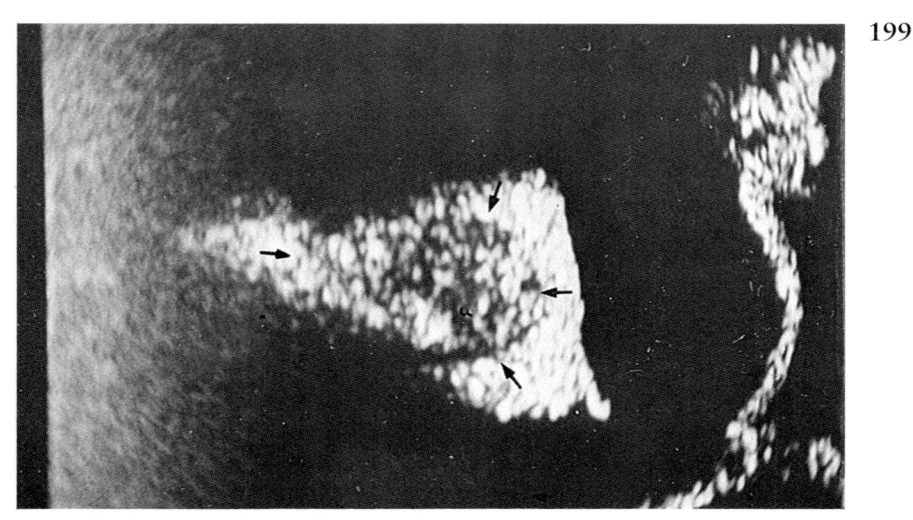

199 Ultrasonography. Orbital cavernous haemangioma (arrows).

Fluorescein angiography of the fundus

Sodium fluorescein solution injected intravenously will rapidly appear in the choroid, the retinal arteries, capillaries and subsequently veins. In the choroid it leaks at once into the extracellular space through the fenestrated endothelium. It does not leak from the retinal vasculature under normal circumstances, as fenestrations are not present in this system. Its appearance is observed and photographed and provides information about posterior segment pathology.

This investigation is probably performed too frequently. It has a definite morbidity and should not be used merely to confirm a diagnosis which is clinically apparent, e.g. if disc new vessels are clearly seen, a fluorescein angiogram is not necessarily required prior to laser therapy. An emergency tray and oxygen should be to hand if fluorescein is to be injected.

Its principal uses are:

>(1) diagnostic, e.g. in ischaemic diabetic maculopathy or in cases where the nature of disc swelling is not clear.
>
>(2) treatment-related, e.g. to demonstrate the site of leak in a central serous retinopathy which fails to resolve spontaneously, or to identify the location of a subretinal neovascular membrane where treatment is contemplated e.g. in early disciform degeneration of the macula.

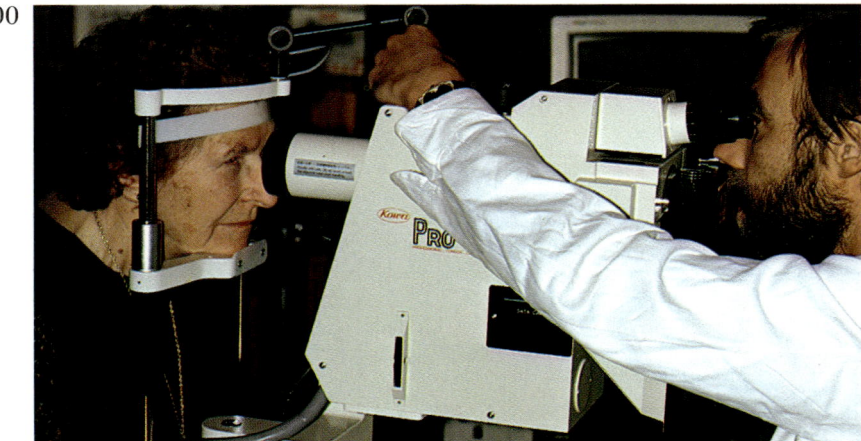

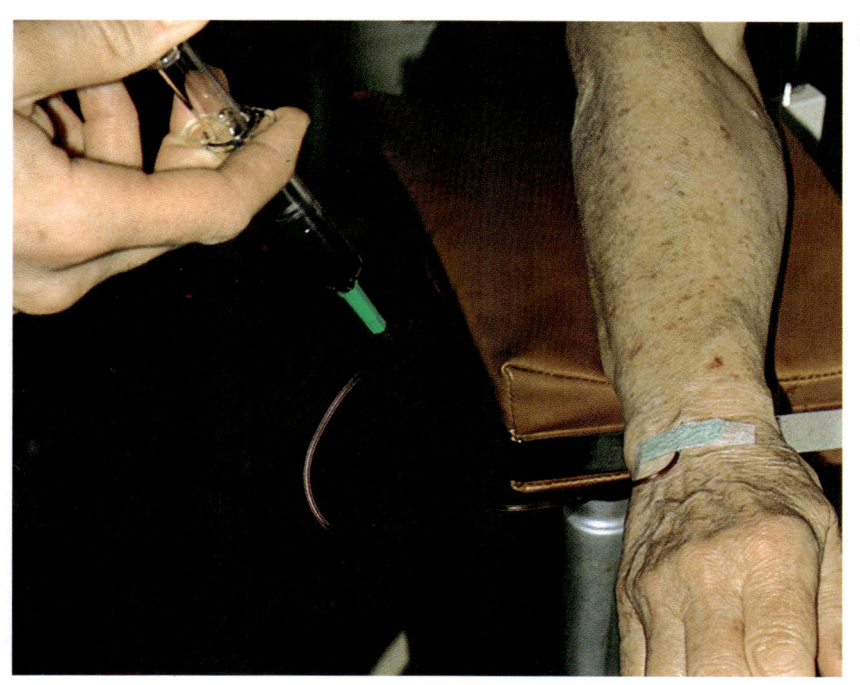

201 Fluorescein angiography. A butterfly cannula is inserted into a vein and a syringe containing 5 ml of 10 or 20 per cent sodium fluorescein is attached. When the posterior pole is in focus the fluorescein is injected in a bolus and a series of photographs at 0.6 to 0.8 second intervals is taken.

200 Fluorescein angiography. The pupils are dilated and the patient is seated at the camera. A repeat-firing fundus camera is required, with interchangeable camera bodies to permit colour photographs to be taken prior to the black and white angiography series. The camera contains two types of filter. White light from the camera passes through a blue (excitation) filter, and enters the eye to excite the fluorescein molecules to a higher wavelength (green). A green (barrier) filter blocks the return of any blue light so that only the green emitted by the fluorescein is recorded on film. A movable target for the patient to watch is used when the periphery is to be photographed.

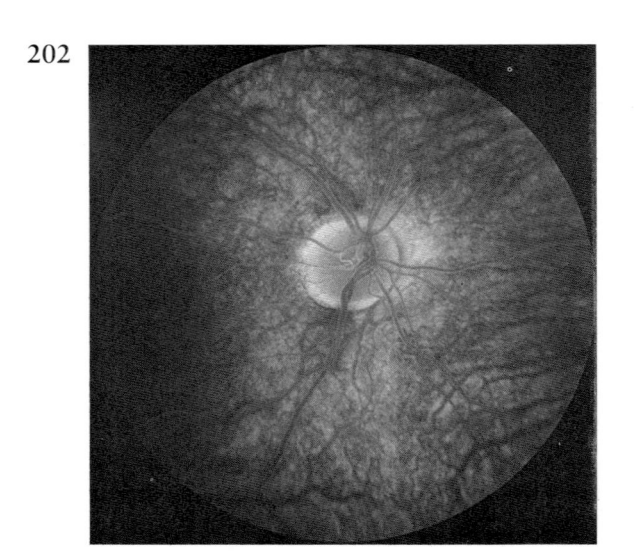

202 Fluorescein angiogram. A normal disc—choroidal filling.

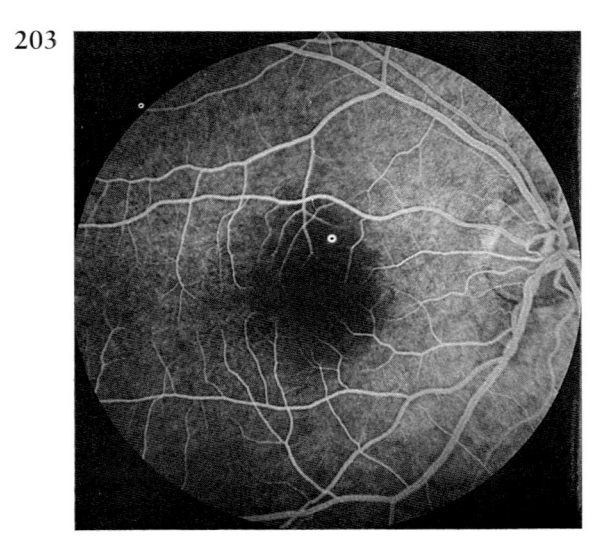

203 Fluorescein angiogram. A normal macula. Dye (white) is seen filling the retinal arteries and veins over the choroidal fluorescence.

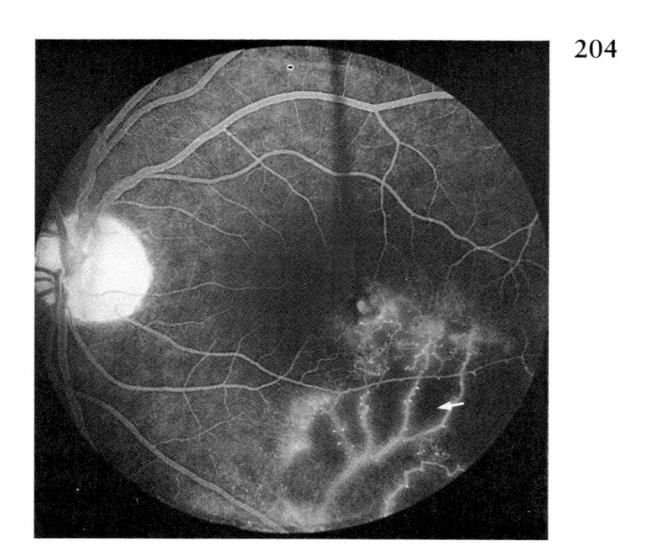

204 Fluorescein angiogram. Area of ischaemic retina (arrow) crossed by abnormal vessels. A vertical fixation pointer identifies the fovea.

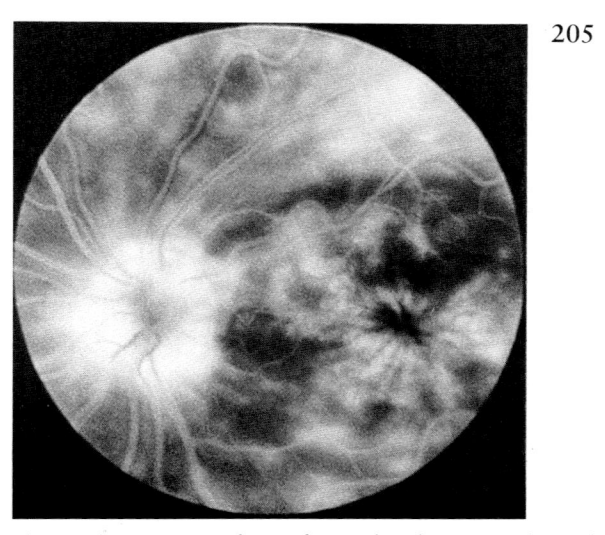

205 Fluorescein angiogram. Leakage from the disc, vessels and macula (cystoid macular oedema). Behçet's disease.

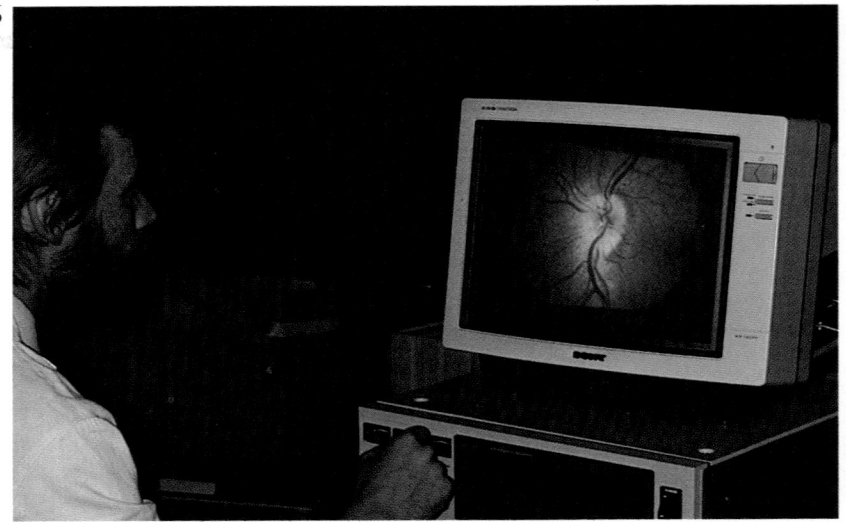

206 Fluorescein angiogram. Video recording has also become available for angiographic studies.

Each fluorescein series is examined for abnormal anatomy, areas of hyperfluorescence (caused by leakage or increased transmission of choroidal fluorescence), and hypofluorescence (filling defects, block of transmission of choroidal fluorescence).

Pseudofluorescence occurs when fluorescence in the media (aqueous or vitreous) is reflected from fundus structures e.g. myelinated nerve fibres.

Autofluorescence is a property of fluorescence of certain tissues or entities, such as drusen of the optic nerve head, and may be seen in red-free photographs (in the absence of injected fluorescein).

11 Tests in ocular injuries

As always, accurate clinical observations take precedence over further tests, e.g. a reduction of intra-ocular pressure, a distorted pupil, a shallowed anterior chamber, are suggestive of ocular penetration.

Seidel's test

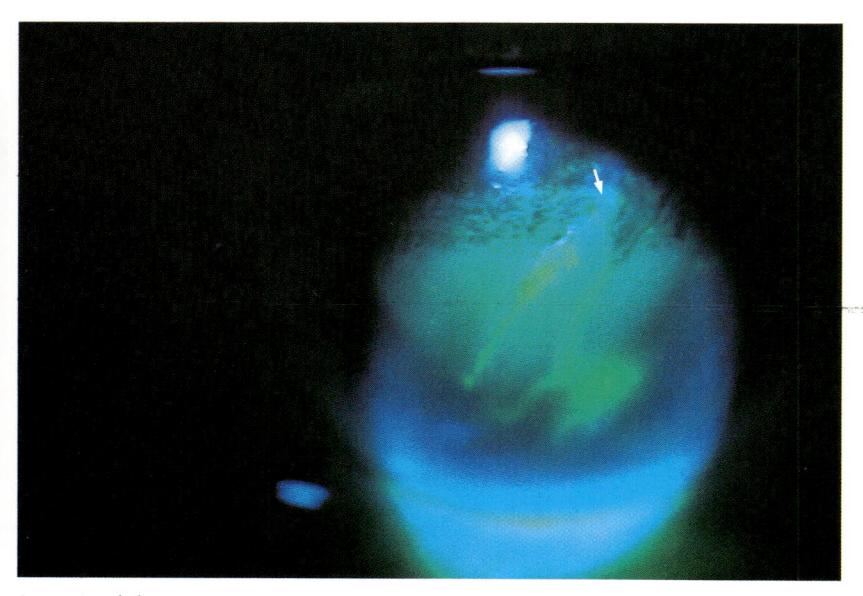

207

207 Seidel's test. Suspected aqueous leak through a corneal injury should be confirmed by applying 2 per cent fluorescein to the superior bulbar conjunctiva and examining under blue light. The fluorescein is diluted by aqueous and forms a conspicuous fluorescent stream running down from the leak (arrow).

Radiology

Plain X-rays are now supplemented by CT scans to elucidate trauma (in addition to ultrasonography, Chapter 10).

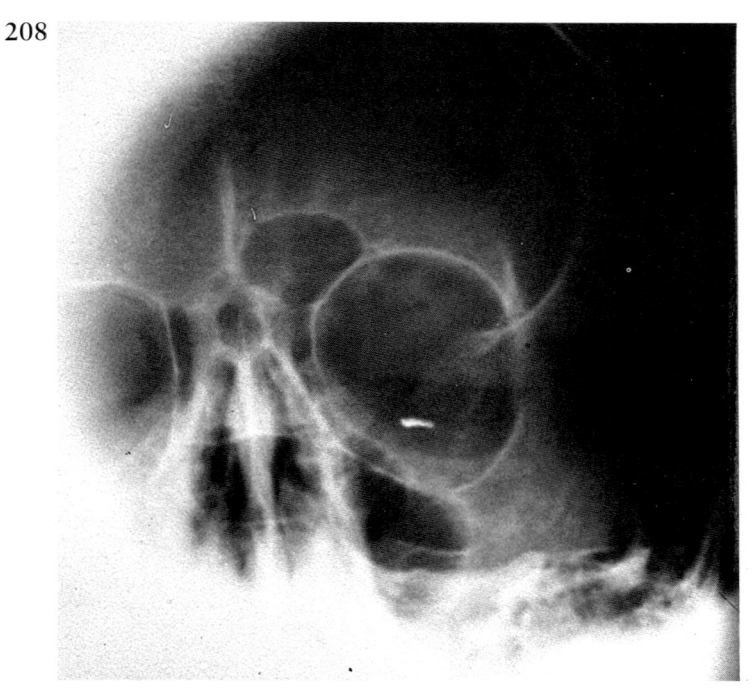

208 Skull X-ray (PA). A metallic foreign body is seen.

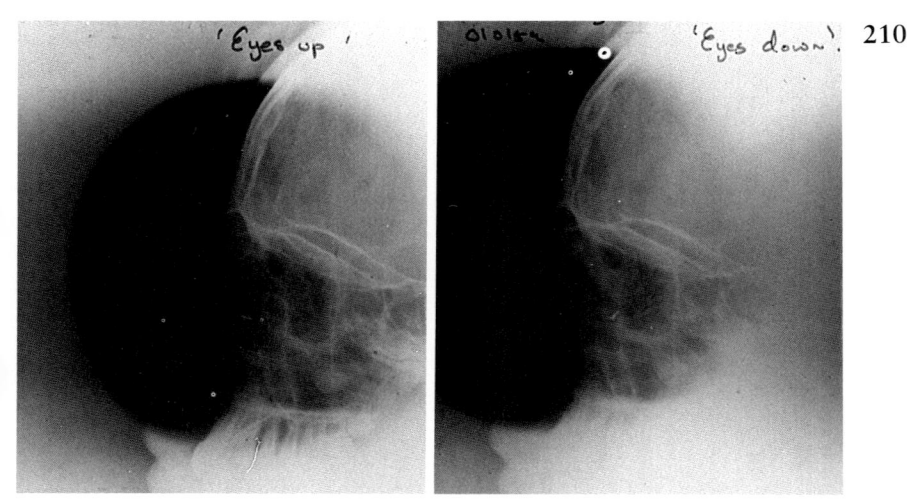

209 and **210 Skull X-rays (lateral).** Looking up (**209**), and looking down (**210**). The foreign body is seen to move with respect to the orbital rim when the eyes move and so is likely to be within the globe.

211 CT scan. A foreign body is seen in the globe (arrow). This is becoming the preferred method of visualization.

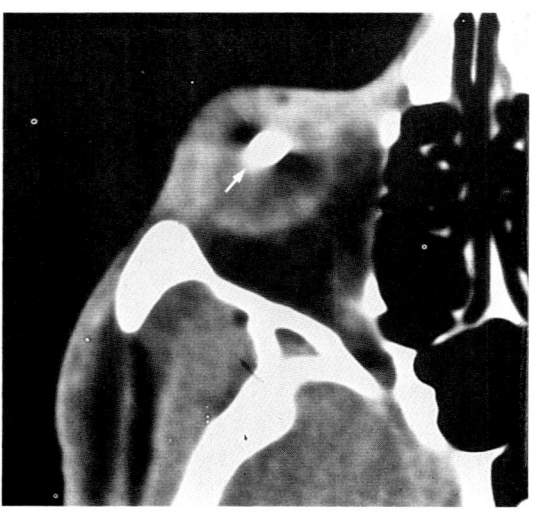

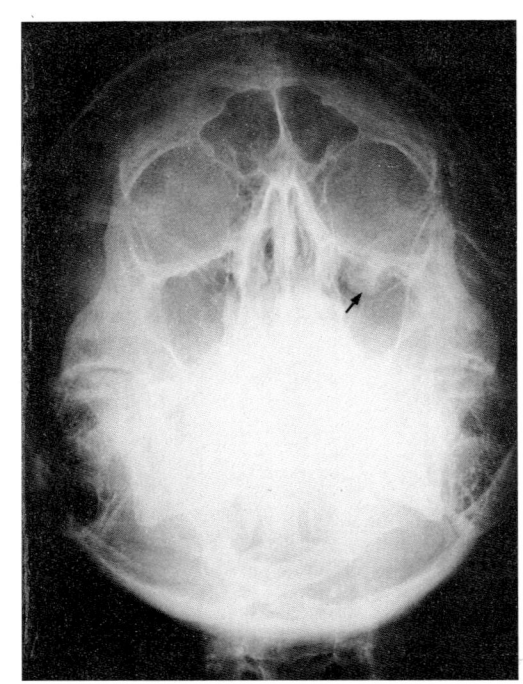

212 Skull X-ray. Blowout fracture of orbit. The prolapsed orbital tissues form a characteristic 'tear drop' in the roof of the maxillary sinus (arrow).

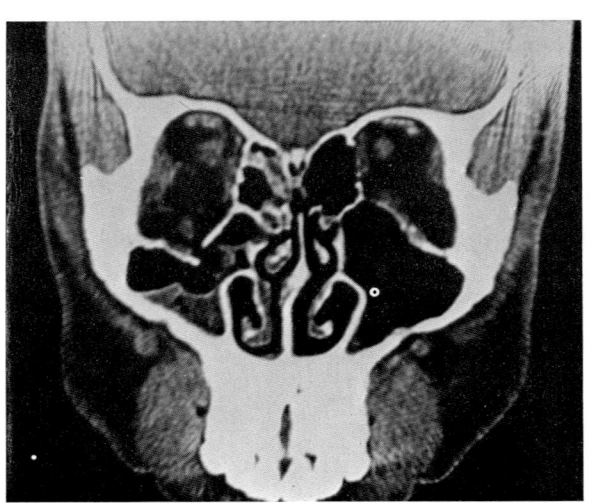

213 CT scan. Orbital blowout fracture (coronal). The fragment is displaced into the right maxillary antrum and an air-fluid interface is seen.

12 Basic tests in optics

The strength of spectacle lenses may be determined by neutralization with lenses of equal but opposite power, or more usually with a focimeter. To achieve the best visual acuity, refraction is performed. Keratometry is required for contact lens practice, and is combined with biometry to select the strength of lens implants.

Neutralization of lenses

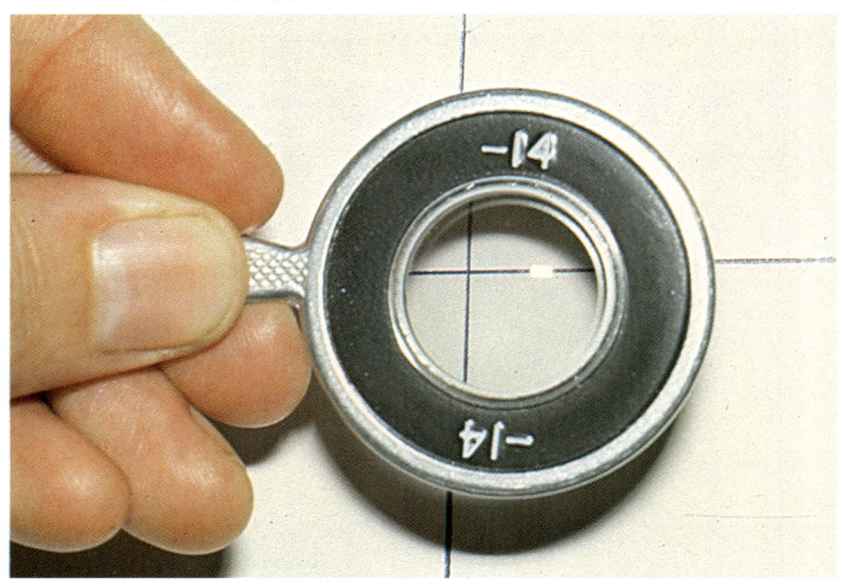

214 Lens type. A cross larger than the lens is drawn on a piece of paper. The lens is held several centimetres above the cross and moved left and right, and up and down to determine its sign. A minus lens will move the centre of the cross in the same direction as the lens movement.

215

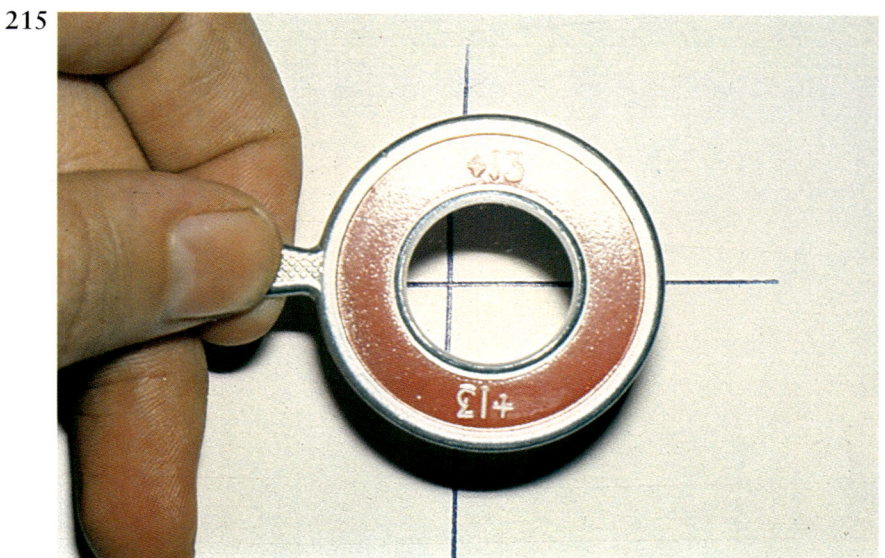

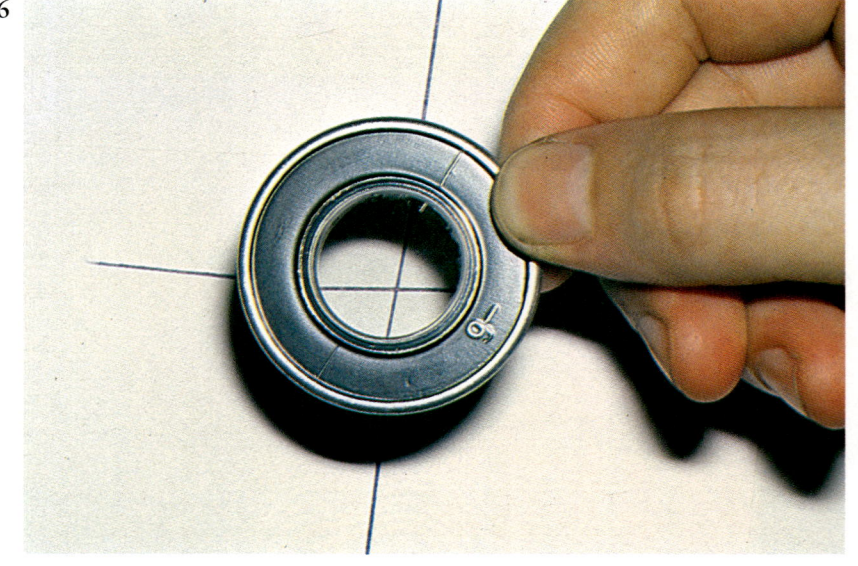

216

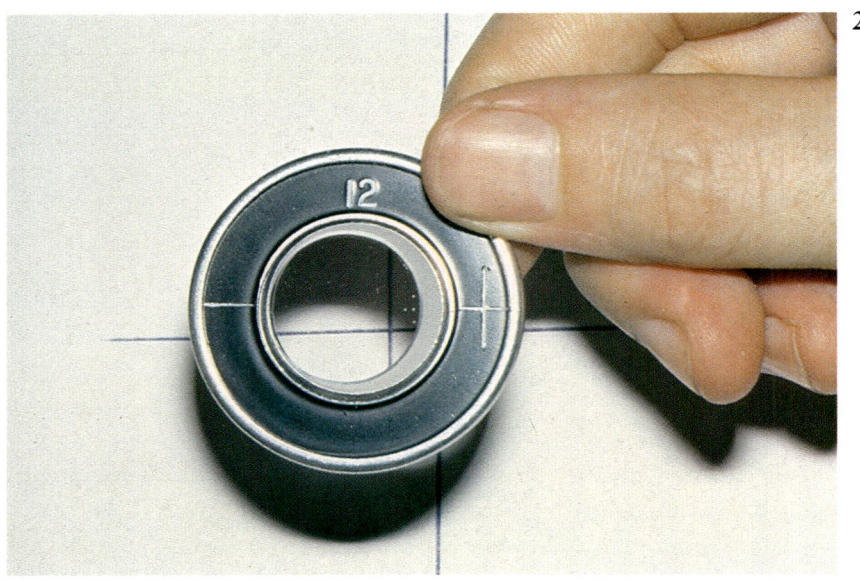

215 Lens type. A plus lens moves the centre of the cross in the opposite direction.

216 Lens type. The lens is then rotated around the centre of the cross. If the cross twists, as shown, there is a cylindrical component to the lens. The lens is then positioned so that the cross is aligned.

217 Lens type. If the centre of the cross is displaced laterally, despite all attempts to centre the cross over it, a prism component exists in the unknown lens.

A lens of the opposite sign to the unknown lens is selected and the two lenses are held together. The horizontal and vertical movement over the cross is repeated; when a spherical lens is fully neutralized by its opposite no movement of the cross occurs. With a spherocylinder, only one axis will be neutralized and the process is then repeated in the other axis.

The focimeter

218

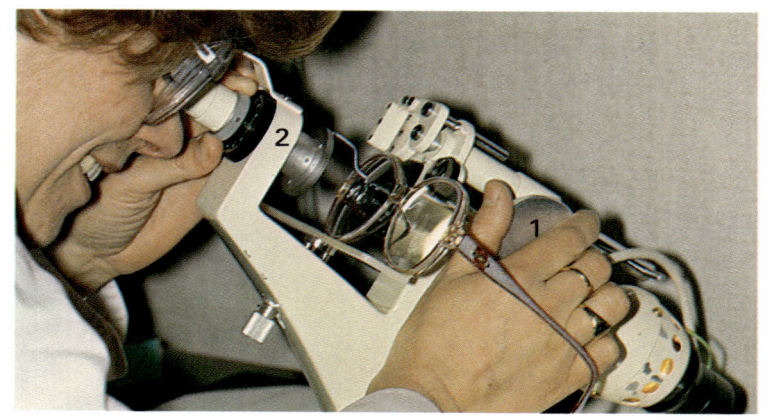

218 Focimeter. The side scale (1) indicates lens power and sign. It is set to 0 dioptres and the eyepiece adjusted until a focussed circle of dots is seen. There is an angular scale (2) which rotates a grid graticule for measuring the axis of cylinders. The spectacles are placed in the instrument facing the examiner (held in place with a rubber-covered support). The right lens is usually measured first.

On looking through the eyepiece, if the dots are still in a circle (though out of focus), the lens is a sphere. The side scale is adjusted until the circle of dots is in focus again and the power noted.

If instead of dots, a set of parallel lines is seen, a cylindrical component is present. The scale is adjusted to focus the lines. The power is noted, e.g. −4.00. The scale is then further rotated until another set of focussed lines appears, at right angles to the first. The difference in scale reading between this and the first reading is the cylindrical power, e.g. if the focimeter scale now reads −6.00 the difference is −2.00.

The two results are recorded with the difference second e.g. −4.00/−2.00. The angle of the second set of parallel lines corresponds to the axis of the cylinder and is measured using the angular scale; the indicator line is exactly aligned with the parallel lines, and the angle is read off the scale in degrees, e.g. 30°. This is the angle of the cylinder (along its axis as decreed by convention). The final result is recorded as −4.00 DS/−2.00 DC × 30. This technique can be practised with a known combination of lenses from a trial set.

Refraction—using a streak retinoscope

A brief description of the basic technique will be given here. Retinoscopy is performed to give an objective refraction. Subjective testing refines this result.

Objective refraction

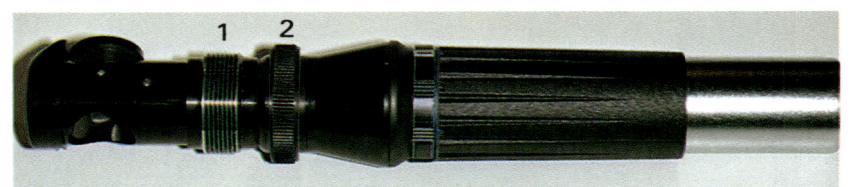

219 Streak retinoscope. The sleeve (1) should be at its lowest point—this controls the relation of the filament and the convex lens within the instrument and at its other extreme the 'with' and 'against' movement of the image will be inverted. The light is switched on and the streak adjusted (2) to a horizontal position.

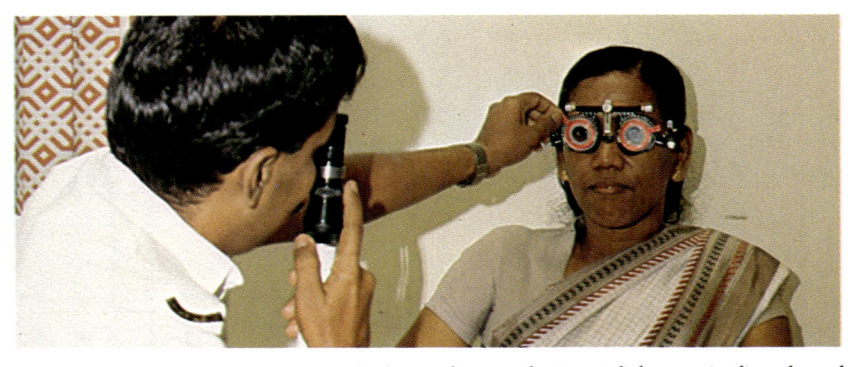

220 Retinoscopy. The room light is dimmed. A trial frame is fitted and the patient is instructed to fix on a distant point, e.g. the chart at 6 m, to avoid accommodation. The examiner sits at a known working distance, commonly ⅔ m from the patient, almost in front of the patient while not blocking his view of the chart, and looks through the retinoscope at the patient's right pupil.

The pupils are not usually dilated. The horizontal streak is shone on the right pupil and moved up and down while the examiner watches the pupil. When he tilts the retinoscope light up, the light seen in the pupil (the reflection from the retina) may move up, i.e. 'with' the retinoscope, or down i.e. 'against' the retinoscope. The rays reflected from the patient's retina are deviated by the optics of the patient's eye and the trial frame lenses and may be divergent, parallel or convergent, as illustrated in **221**.

Parallel and divergent rays produce a 'with' movement (**221**, 1 and 2). Convergent rays produce:

> a) a 'with' movement if the focal point is behind the observer, as occurs in myopia less negative than the reciprocal of the working distance (**221**, 3), i.e. between 0 and -1.5 DS,
>
> b) no movement if focussed at the observer, as occurs in myopia equal to the reciprocal of the working distance (**221**, 4), i.e. -1.5 DS,
>
> c) an 'against' movement if focussed between the patient and the observer, as occurs in a myopia more negative than the reciprocal of the working distance (**221**, 5), i.e. more negative than -1.5 DS, for a working distance of $2/3$ m.

A lens of the appropriate sign and low strength, e.g. $+0.25$ DS for a 'with' movement, is inserted into the trial frame on the right. The process is repeated. If the movement is still 'with', a stronger lens e.g. $+0.50$ DS is inserted and the first lens removed. This continues until the movement changes to the opposite type e.g. the 'with' becomes 'against'. As soon as that reversal is reached the refractive error has been corrected in that meridian for that working distance.

221 The optics of retinoscopy. The observer's and subject's eyes are represented by retinal planes (Ro, Rs), principal (pupillary) planes (Ho, Hs) and nodal points (No, Ns). The retinoscope light is moved from the common optical axis (NoNs) in the direction indicated by the arrow on the subject's retinal plane. The rays emerging from the illuminated area of the retina at the arrow tip are illustrated. An image is formed at I. A line drawn from I through the observer's nodal point indicates the way the observer perceives the image. The curved arrows show the direction of movement seen by the observer.

THE OPTICS OF RETINOSCOPY

1 Emmetropia   Working distance ⅔m

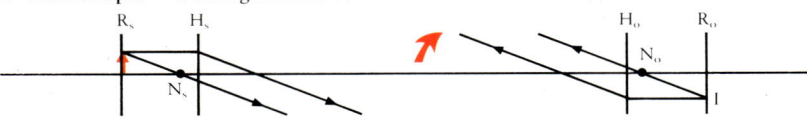

The emerging rays are parallel. A 'with' movement occurs.

2 Hypermetropia

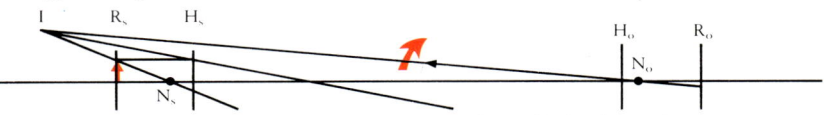

The emerging rays are divergent. A virtual image 'I' is formed behind the subject's eye. A 'with' movement occurs.

3 Myopia 0 to -1.5D

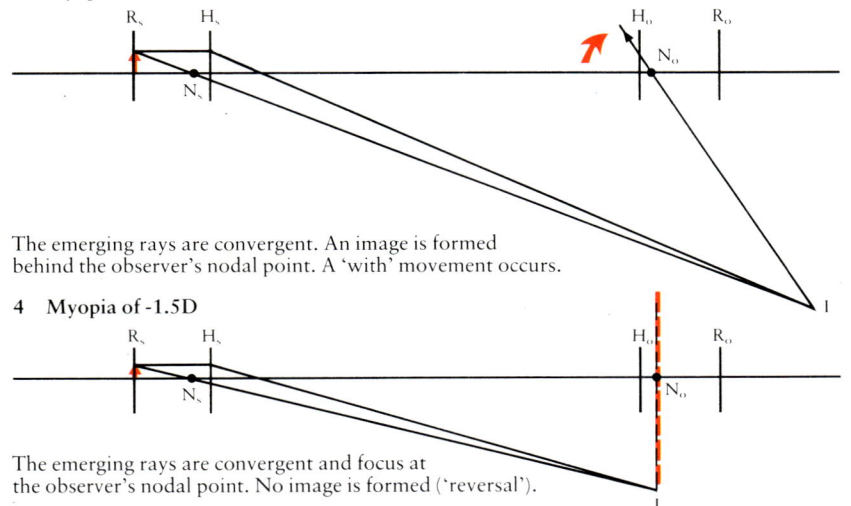

The emerging rays are convergent. An image is formed behind the observer's nodal point. A 'with' movement occurs.

4 Myopia of -1.5D

The emerging rays are convergent and focus at the observer's nodal point. No image is formed ('reversal').

5 Myopia of more than -1.5D

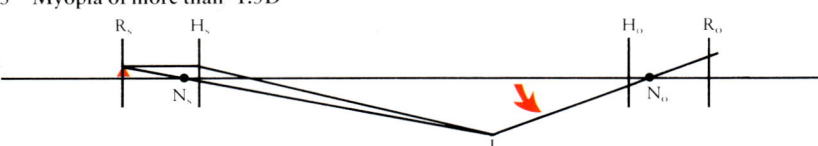

Emerging rays are convergent. The image is formed in front of the observer's nodal point. An 'against' movement occurs.

Simultaneously, the horizontal meridian is examined with a vertical streak and a right-left movement, and the results recorded as the objective refraction, for example:

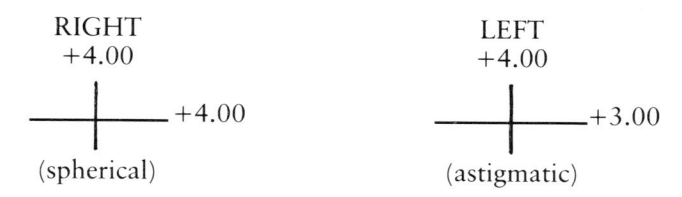

RIGHT
+4.00

——┼—— +4.00

(spherical)

LEFT
+4.00

——┼——+3.00

(astigmatic)

To obtain the correction for infinity the reciprocal of the working distance is subtracted e.g. if +4.00 DS results in reversal, the patient's error is +2.50 DS (at a working distance of ⅔ m, 1.5 is subtracted).

If the patient has only a spherical error both the vertical and horizontal meridia will be the same. If the reversal point is reached at a different strength of lens in each meridian, the patient is astigmatic, i.e. requires a cylindrical correction.

If the reflex seen in the pupil is not parallel to the streak input, this indicates that the patient is astigmatic and the axis of the correction is not along the vertical or horizontal meridian. The process described above is carried out but the streak input is directed along that axis in which parallel reflection occurs and at right angles to it. The angles are noted and the astigmatism described accordingly.

When some facility has been achieved with the above, the two eyes may be refracted simultaneously, i.e. increasing the strength of lenses in both eyes and observing the movement of the streak in each meridian of first the right then the left eye. This has the advantage of speed, and prevents errors due to accommodation of the uncovered eye as hypermetropia is corrected.

If no clear reflex is seen initially, either the media are cloudy, or the patient has a very large error, e.g. −14.00 DS. A high positive and high negative lens e.g. +10.00 DS and −10.00 DS should be tried.

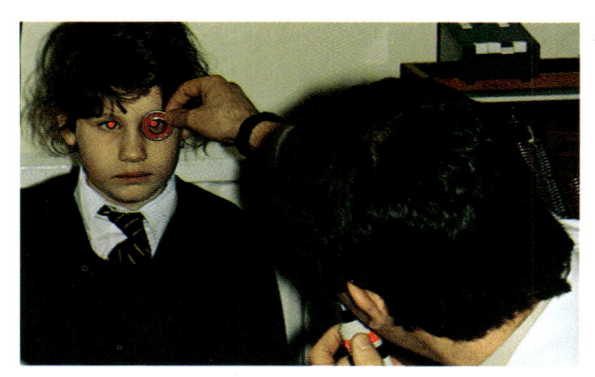

222 Cycloplegic retinoscopy. Children accommodate during refraction and this can be overcome using a cycloplegic e.g. 1 per cent cyclopentolate (after 30-60 minutes) or 1 per cent atropine (after 45 to 80 minutes).

Subjective refraction

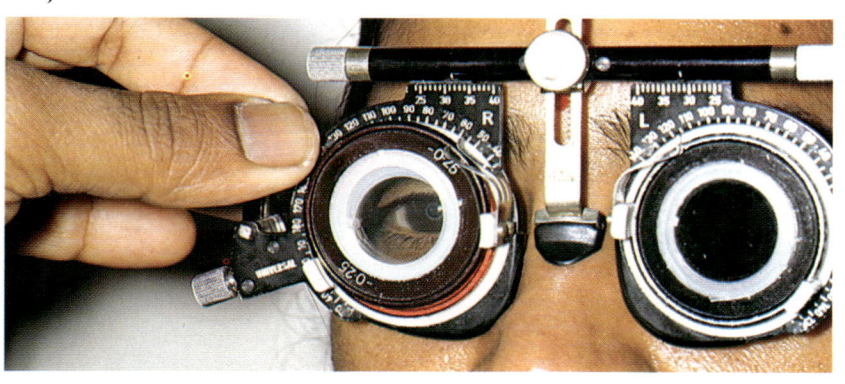

223 Strength of sphere. The correction obtained from retinoscopy minus the inverse of the working distance is inserted in the trial frame for both eyes. One eye is occluded and the patient asked to read the chart, which he should be able to do if the objective refraction is within range, and there is no marked ocular pathology. Minor changes in spherical lens power are then made: +0.25 DS or −0.25 DS is added and enquiry is made regarding improvement.

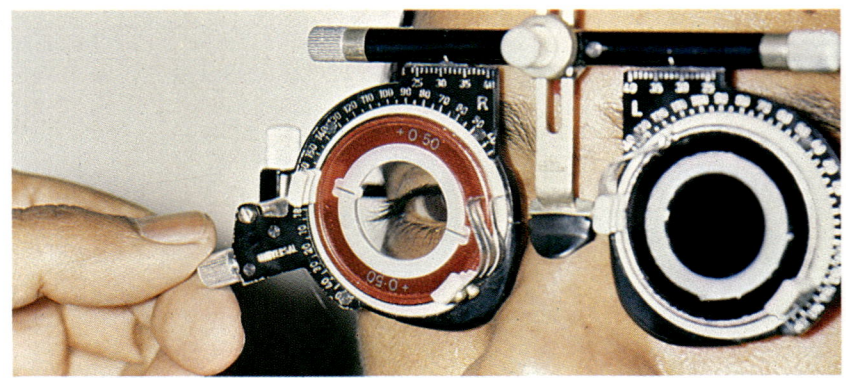

224 Cylinder axis and strength. In astigmatic cases, the cylinder axis is then checked. This can be done by 'spinning' the cylinder as shown, i.e. rotating in 5° steps either way to find the angle that the patient prefers. The strength is verified in the same way as for the sphere, by increasing or decreasing the existing cylinder by 0.25 D in the same axis and asking the patient whether his vision is improved or not.

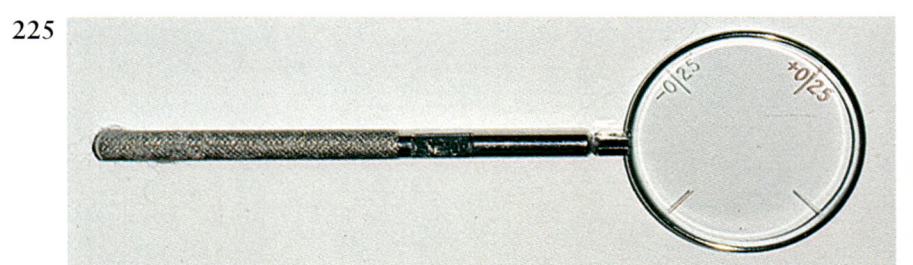

225 The crossed cylinder. An alternative way of checking the cylinder axis and strength is with the crossed cylinder, in which the cylindrical component is twice the power of the spherical component and of opposite sign, e.g. a -0.25 D sphere with a $+0.5$ D cylinder.

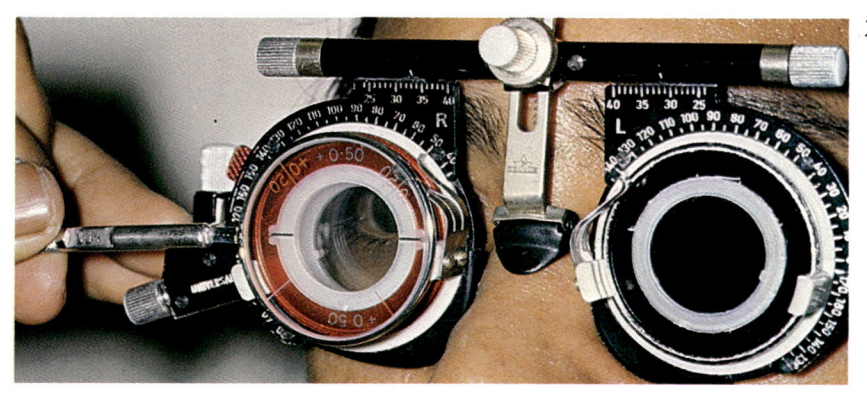

226 The crossed cylinder. The axis of the correcting cylinder is checked by aligning the handle of the crossed cylinder with the axis (as shown), then flipping the lens back and forth. If vision with one position is better than vision with the other, the correcting cylinder is turned 5° in the direction of the crossed cylinder axis marked with the same sign as the lens in question. This is repeated until no change is seen.

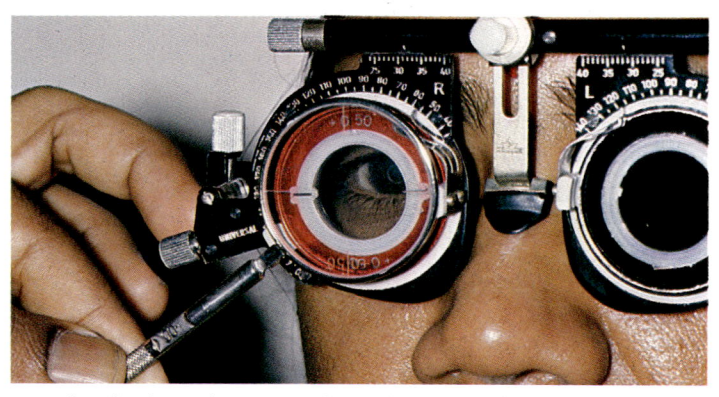

227 The crossed cylinder. The strength is checked by placing each axis of the crossed cylinder in turn over the axis of the correcting cylinder (by placing the handle of the crossed cylinder oblique to the axis as shown and flipping the lens back and forth). If either position improves the vision, a small cylinder of the same sign is added and the process repeated. The final acuity with the best combination of lenses is recorded.

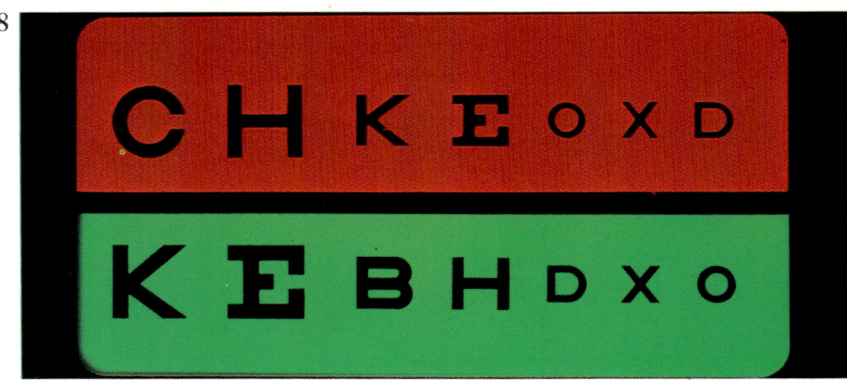

228 The duochrome. Myopes should be corrected so that the red section of the duochrome is just clearer than the green—then they are not overcorrected.

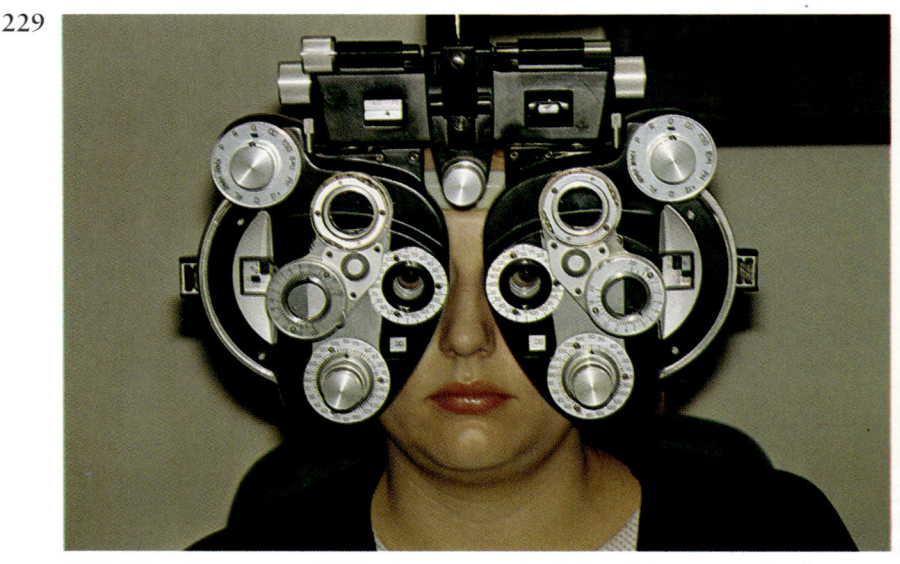

229 The phoropter. All the lenses required for objective and subjective refraction may be incorporated in a single device which is suspended before the patient. This avoids the handling and smearing of desk lens sets. It is not appropriate for testing reading vision.

Near vision
When the patient has been corrected to emmetropia, the near (reading) vision is tested wearing that correction. Patients under 40 years of age without ocular pathology (having adequate accommodation) should be able to read the smallest print in the near vision chart at their usual working distance (usually 30 cm). Patients over 40 generally require an added plus lens to read with ease. In practice, about 0.5 dioptres need to be added for every five years, so a 65-year-old may need an extra +2.5 D before each eye. Overcorrection should be avoided; the patient should still be able to read the chart 12 to 15 cm beyond her working distance.

Separation of visual axes
After the required corrections for distance and near have been determined, the distance between the visual axes must be measured to permit the optician to centre the lenses accurately before the eyes. This is often termed the interpupillary distance, though the visual axis may not go through the centre of the pupil and so they may not be exactly the same.

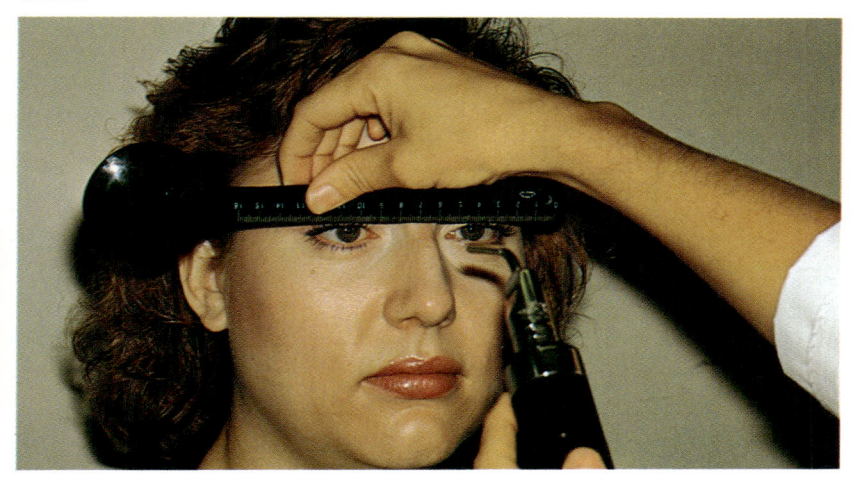

230 Separation of visual axes. The examiner sits facing the patient and holds a light before the right eye. A millimetre ruler is placed on the bridge of the nose with a convenient mark, e.g. 10 mm, over the corneal reflex of the right eye (as seen with the examiner's left eye). The light is then placed before the left eye and the reading on the ruler above the left corneal reflex noted (with the examiner's right eye). The difference in the readings is the required figure.

Centration
The optical centre of a lens is the point through which all rays pass undeviated. It can be located by centering the lens on the focimeter and marking the central point. The distance between the optical centres of lenses in a spectacle frame should correspond to the separation of the patient's visual axes.

Rays that do not pass through the optical centre of the lens are deviated as by a prism, the amount depending on the lens strength. Therefore if centration is inaccurate or the lenses are very different in power, the patient may experience double vision. Alternatively, the spectacle lenses may deliberately be decentred to provide a prismatic effect, for example, to reduce the amount of convergence necessary for near vision.

The geometric centre of a lens is simply the middle point of the spectacle frame.

Phorias in refraction
Most phorias (latent squints) are asymptomatic and so do not require treatment. Symptomatic phorias can be investigated in the refraction context by performing the alternate cover test (Chapter 5) wearing the distance correction, then using the Maddox rod for distance and the Maddox wing for near. With these devices, the image presented to each eye is different, dissociation occurs and the eye takes up the position of rest, at which the deviation is measured.

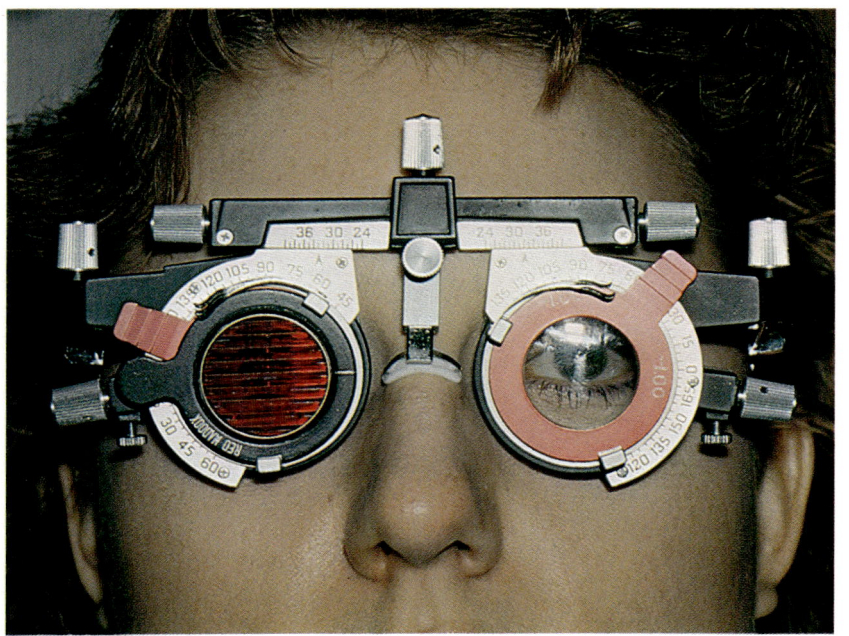

231 Maddox rod. This series of red cylinders makes a white spot look like a red line running perpendicular to the direction of the cylinders. It is placed horizontally before the right eye, a spot of light at 6 m (usually part of the test types box) is fixed upon, and the patient is asked whether the vertical red line (seen by the right eye) runs through the light (seen by the left eye) or beside it.

In orthophoria, the line runs through the light. In esophoria the line will be seen on the right of the light, and vice versa for exophoria. The amount of the phoria is determined by placing prisms horizontally in the trial frame until the line runs through the light. The rod is then placed vertically in the right frame; if there is a right hyperphoria, the horizontal red line will appear below the light, whereas in a left hyperphoria the line appears above the light. The amount is then also measured with additional prisms.

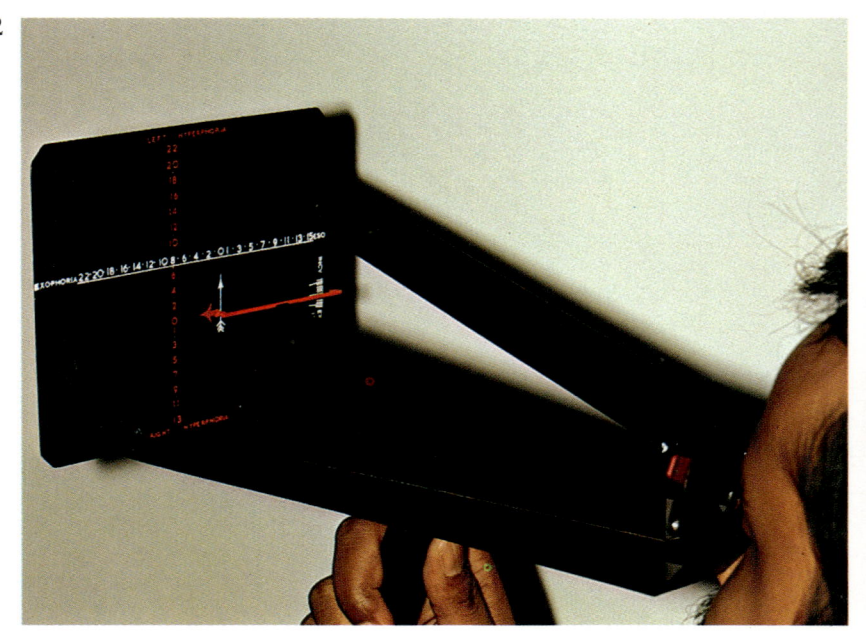

232 Maddox wing. The patient looks through the apertures and sees a vertical and horizontal scale with the left eye and a red and white arrow with the right eye. The field of each eye is separated from the other by septa. The readings on the scale as seen by the patient correspond to the amount of vertical and horizontal deviation.

Keratometry

This is the measurement of the curvature of the anterior corneal surface. The cornea acts as a convex mirror and the greater the curvature of the mirror the smaller the reflected image. The magnification produced by the reflector is the ratio of image size to object size. Either the image size is kept constant and the object size varied, as in the instrument shown, or vice versa. Illuminated mires form the object used to produce the reflected image.

233 Keratometer (Javal-Schiotz type). The mires are shown.

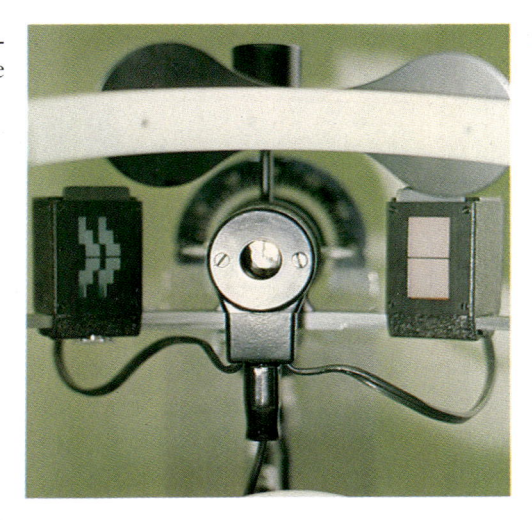

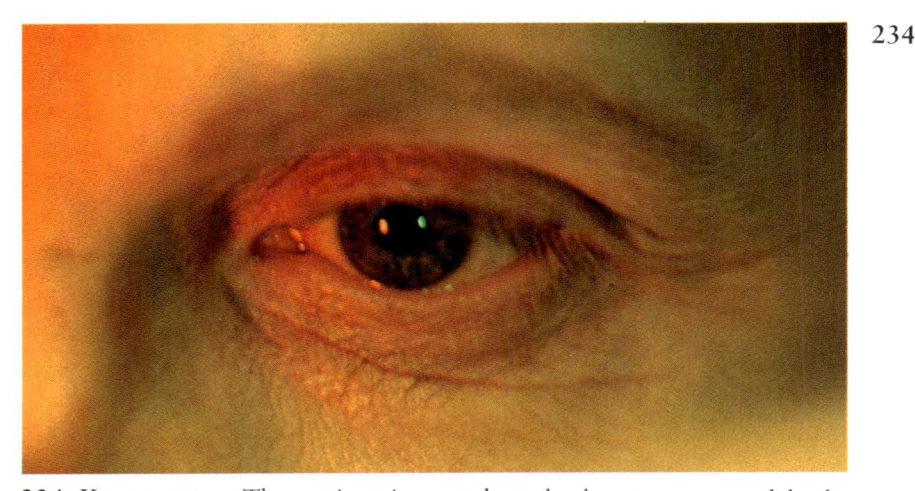

234 Keratometry. The patient is seated at the keratometer and looks straight ahead. The examiner observes the reflection of the mires in the cornea (illustrated) and adjusts the mires to the endpoint shown in **235**. The radius of curvature and the dioptric power in that meridian can be read off the scale. The frame supporting the mires is then rotated through 90° and another reading taken.

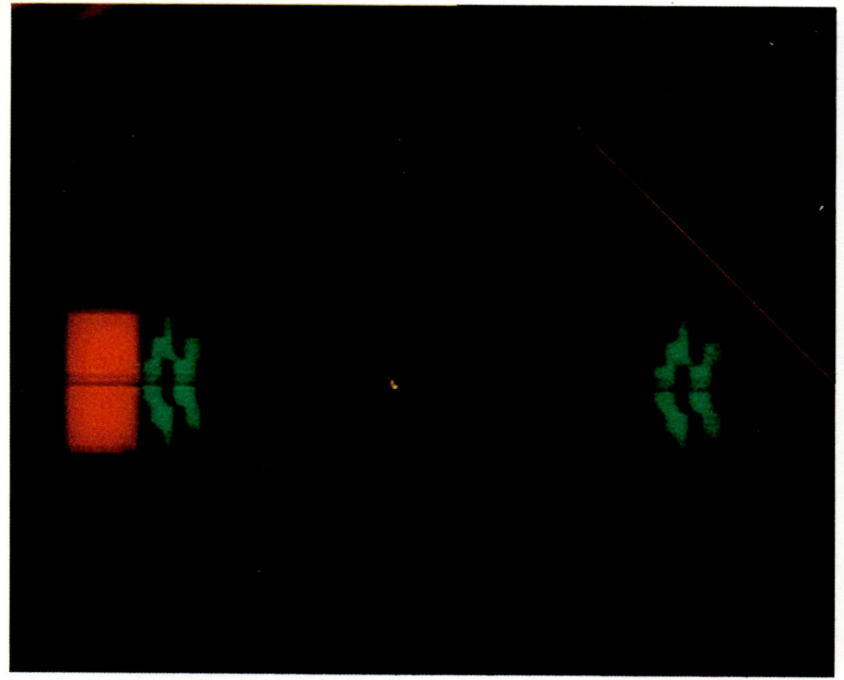

235 Keratometry. Endpoint of adjustment of mires, seen through the eye piece. The image is doubled by a prism to overcome the problem of eye movements interfering with measurement. If an oblique astigmatism were present, the lines bisecting both sets of mires would not be aligned and the instrument would have to be rotated until they were aligned prior to taking the reading. The angle of the astigmatism could then be read off the scale.

Biometry

Prior to insertion of an intra-ocular lens, the patient's corneal curvature is determined by keratometry and the axial length of the eye by ultrasound biometry. The two results are combined with a figure for the presumed intra-ocular lens plane in a formula to calculate the required strength of the lens.

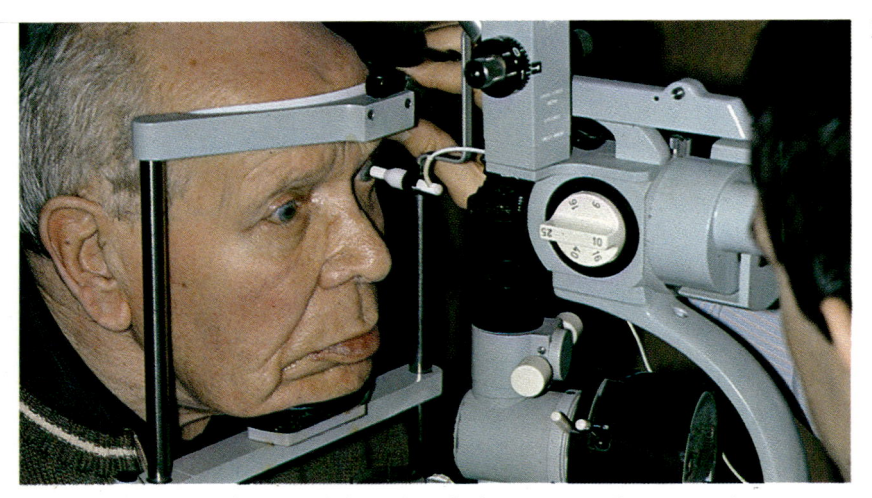

236 Biometry. The axial length of the eye is determined using an ultrasound transducer which can be applied to the cornea, which is anaesthetized.

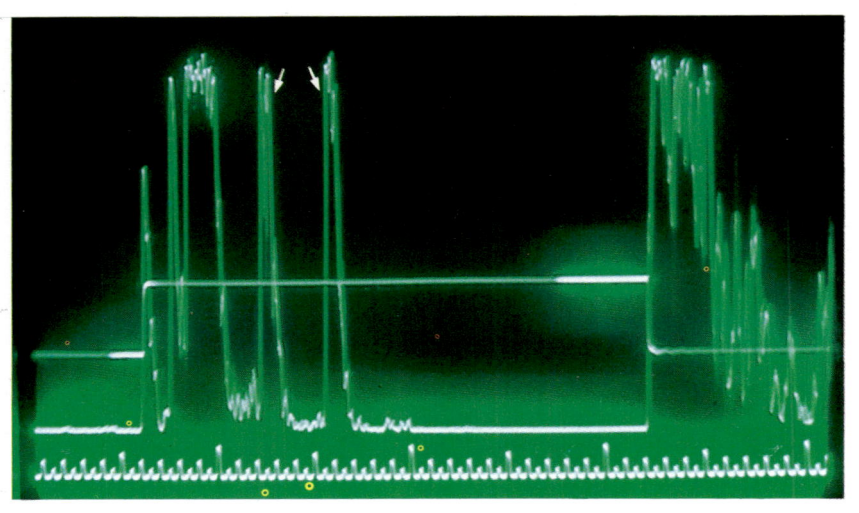

237 Biometry. The reading is in the linear A mode. The reflections from the cornea, lens (arrows), and fundus are seen.

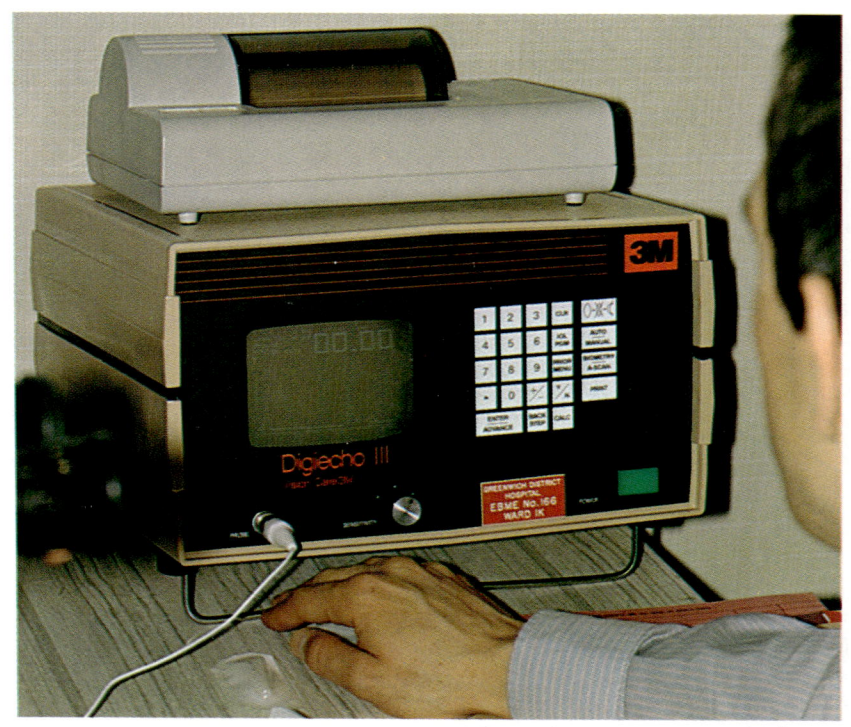

238 Biometry. The axial length is read from the instrument, which can also be used to calculate the intra-ocular lens power required.

13 Tests for systemic disease

Systemic diseases involving the eye are principally vascular, inflammatory, or neoplastic (including reticulo-endothelial neoplasms). With all ocular disorders the possibility of a systemic link should be considered.

Diabetes and hypertension are so common, and diabetes in particular is linked with such a multitude of ocular changes, that ideally all new patients should have their blood pressure taken and their urine or blood sugar tested.

Subsequent to the clinical examination it is usual to consider further investigations in the subgroups of:

    Blood tests
    Skin tests e.g. Mantoux, Kveim
    Radiology
    'Special tests' e.g. the Tensilon test, electromyography, bone marrow biopsy, etc.

The 'special tests' may be undertaken in cooperation with neurologists or other physicians. Temporal artery biopsy will be described in detail because it is usually performed by ophthalmologists.

Ocular abnormality	*Relevant tests.*
Variable ptosis or diplopia	Tensilon test, electromyography, acetylcholine receptor antibodies, mediastinal CT scan for thymoma (myasthenia gravis).
Proptosis	Haemoglobin, white blood cell count, ESR (cellulitis, lymphoproliferative disorders, granulomas), blood sugar (cellulitis or mucormycosis in diabetics), T4, T3, TRH test, (thyrotoxicosis), VDRL, FTA, TPHA (syphilitic gumma), Mantoux (tuberculoma), chest X-ray (primary neoplasm, granuloma), skull X-rays, orbital X-rays, CT scans.

Ocular palsy	Blood pressure (hypertension), haemoglobin, ESR (vasculitis, e.g. temporal arteritis, sarcoidosis, polyarteritis nodosa, systemic lupus erythematosus), blood sugar (diabetic infarct), VDRL (syphilitic gumma or vasculitis), radiology as for proptosis.
Dry eyes, scleritis	Rheumatoid factor (rheumatoid arthritis).
Uveitis	VDRL, ESR (auto-immune disorders), Mantoux, Kveim (sarcoidosis), chest X-ray (sarcoidosis, Wegener's), sacro-iliac joint X-ray (ankylosing spondylitis). (Anterior uveitis is common and tests other than the VDRL are only performed where suggestive symptoms exist. In posterior uveitis and vasculitis the diagnosis must often be made on clinical grounds, e.g. Behçet's disease.)
Retinal emboli	Examination for carotid bruit and cardiac murmurs, blood pressure and blood sugar (causes of arteriopathy), electrocardiography (atrial fibrillation), echocardiography (valve disease), chest X-ray (large left atrium, calcified valves), venous subtraction scans and Doppler studies (carotid stenosis).
Retinal vein occlusions and haemorrhages	Haemoglobin (polycythaemia, anaemia), ESR (hyperviscosity syndromes, e.g. multiple myeloma), blood pressure and blood sugar, VDRL.
Anterior ischaemic optic neuropathy	ESR (giant cell arteritis), blood pressure and blood sugar, temporal artery biopsy (giant cell arteritis).
Cotton wool spots	Blood pressure, blood sugar, haemoglobin, ESR, anti-HIV (AIDS) antibodies.

Temporal artery biopsy

239 Giant cell arteritis. The anterior branch of the superficial temporal artery arises 5 cm above the posterior root of the zygomatic arch and runs tortuously upwards and forwards towards the tuberosity of the frontal bone. If giant cell arteritis is suspected on clinical grounds, treatment must begin immediately. The artery biopsy is performed within 48 hours.

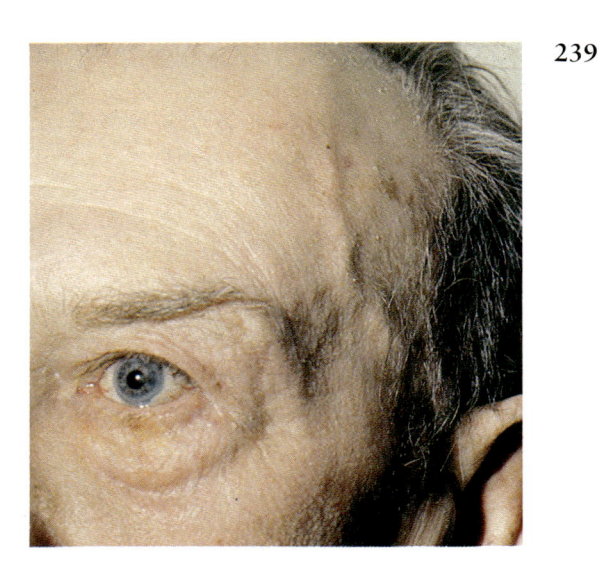

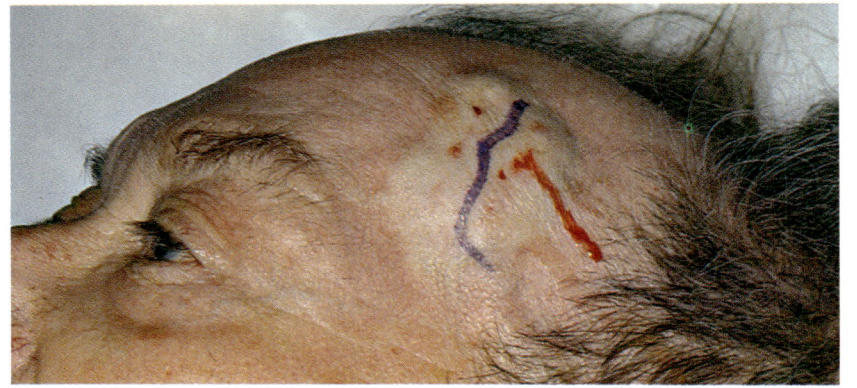

240 Temporal artery biopsy. The procedure is performed in the operating theatre using standard sterile technique. The artery is located, marked and local anaesthetic is infiltrated e.g. 1 per cent lignocaine with adrenaline 1 in 200,000 to reduce bleeding (dose related to age, size and cardiovascular status of patient).

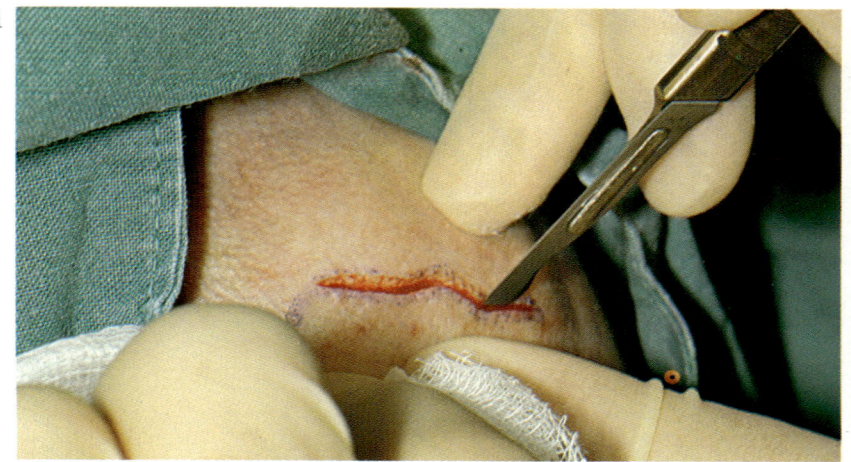

241 Temporal artery biopsy. An incision is made through the skin and fascia over the artery with a scalpel.

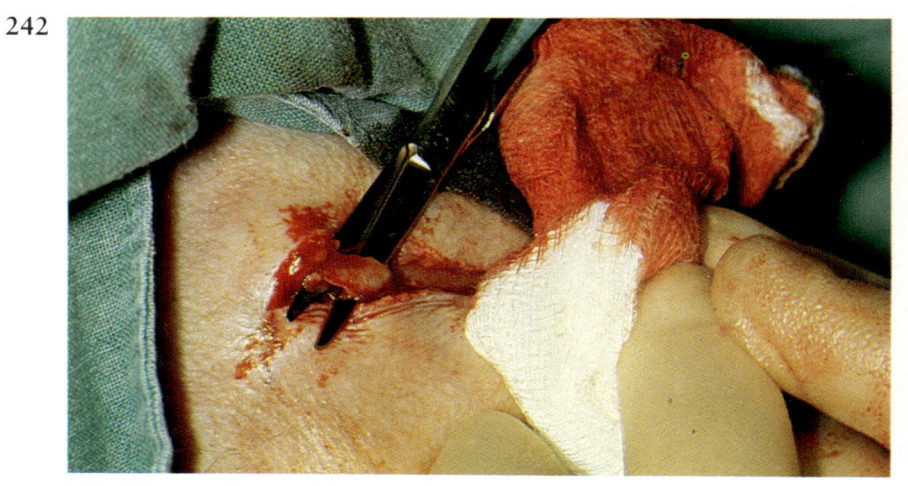

242 Temporal artery biopsy. The artery is dissected out with scissors.

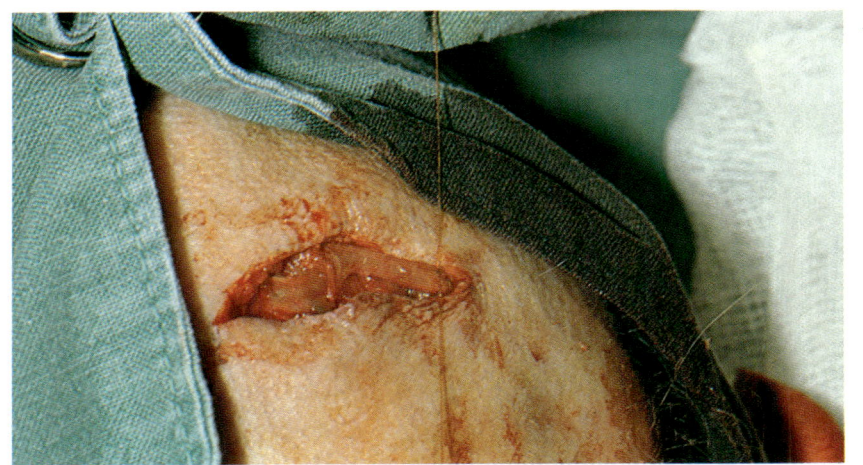

243 Temporal artery biopsy. The artery is ligated twice either side of the planned site of biopsy. These ties must be tight and reliable.

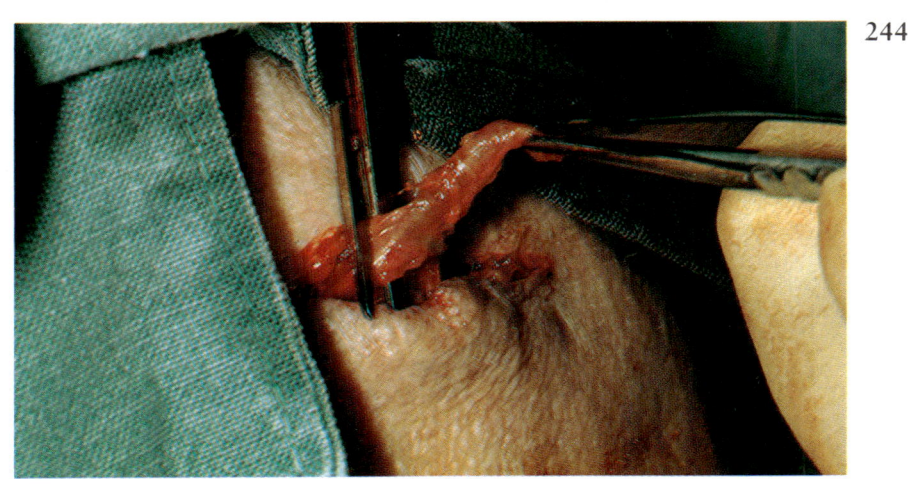

244 Temporal artery biopsy. At least 2 cm of artery are removed if possible, cutting between the ties. The specimen is placed in formol saline and labelled for transfer to the pathology laboratory. The wound is closed and dressed.

References

Chapter 2

Cashell GTW, Durran IM. *Handbook of Orthoptic Principles*, 4th ed. Edinburgh: Churchill Livingstone, 1980.

Duke-Elder S. *Practice of Refraction*, 9th ed. Edinburgh: Churchill Livingstone, 1978.

Hoyt CS, Nickel BL, Billson FA. Ophthalmological Examination of the Infant. Developmental Aspects. *Surv Ophthalmol* 1982; 264: 177-189.

Pelli DG, Robson JG, Wilkins AJ. The design of a new letter chart for measuring contrast sensitivity. *Clin Vision Sci* 1988; 2: 3: 187-199.

Chapter 3

Bron AJ, McKenzie PJ. Ocular anaesthesia. In: Rice AT, Michels RG, Stark WJ. *Rob & Smith's Operative Surgery, Ophthalmic Surgery*, 4th ed. London: Butterworths, 1984.

Duke-Elder WS. *Textbook of Ophthalmology*, Vol. II. p 1128. St Louis: CV Mosby, 1938.

Harley RD. *Paediatric Ophthalmology*, 2nd ed, Vol 1. Philadelphia: WB Saunders, 1983.

Chapter 4

Collin JRO. *A Manual of Systematic Eyelid Surgery*. Edinburgh: Churchill Livingstone, 1983.

Duke-Elder S. *System of Ophthalmology, Vol XII*, Chapter X, p 717, *Ocular dissociations*. St Louis: CV Mosby, 1971.

Fishman G. Hereditary Retinal and Choroidal Diseases: Electroretinogram and Electro-oculogram Findings. In: Peyman GA, Sanders DR, Goldberg MF. *Principles and Practice of Ophthalmology*, Vol 2, Chapter 13. Philadelphia: WB Saunders, 1980.

Glaser JS. Neuro-ophthalmologic examination: General Considerations and Special Techniques. In: Duane TD, ed. *Clinical Ophthalmology*, Vol 2, Chapter 2. Philadelphia: Harper & Row, 1983.

Gonzalez CF, Becker MH, Flanagan JC. *Diagnostic Imaging in Ophthalmology.* New York: Springer Verlag, 1986.

Halliday AM, McDonald WI, Mushin J. Delayed Visual Evoked Response in Optic Neuritis. *Lancet* 1972; 1: 982.

Leigh RJ, Zee DS. *The Neurology of Eye Movements.* Philadelphia: FA Davis, 1983.

Levatin P. Pupillary Escape in Disease of the Retina or Optic Nerve. *Arch Ophthalmol* 1959; 62: 768.

Miller NR. *Walsh & Hoyt's Clinical Neuroophthalmology*, 4th ed., Vol 2, Chapter 40. Baltimore: The Williams and Wilkins Company, 1985.

Musch DC, Frueh BR, Landis JR. The Reliability of Hertel Exophthalmometry. *Ophthalmology* 1985; 92: 1177.

Rothman SLG. Radiology. In: Walsh TJ. *Neuro-Ophthalmology: Clinical Signs and Symptoms*, 2nd ed., Chapter 8. Philadelphia: Lea & Febiger, 1985.

Trobe JD, Ascosta PC, Krischer JP, Trick GL. Confrontation Visual Field Techniques in the Detection of Anterior Visual Pathway Lesions. *Ann Neurol* 1981; 10: 28-34.

Trobe JD, Glaser JS. *The Visual Fields Manual.* Gainesville Florida: Triad Publishing Company, 1983.

Walsh TJ. Ptosis. In: Walsh TJ. *Neuro-ophthalmology: Clinical Signs and Symptoms*, 2nd ed., Chapter 5. Philadelphia: Lea & Febiger, 1985.

Wright JE, Fells P, Jones BR. The Investigation of Proptosis. *Trans Ophthalmol Soc UK* 1970; 90: 221.

Chapter 5

Cashell GTW, Durran IM. *Handbook of Orthoptic Principles.* Edinburgh: Churchill Livingstone, 1980.

Parks, MM. Single Binocular Vision. In: Duane TD, ed. *Clinical Ophthalmology*, Vol 1, Chapter 5. Hagerstown MD: Harper and Row, 1983.

Romano PE, Von Noorden GK. Atypical Responses to the Four-diopter Prism Test. *Amer J. Ophthalmol* 1969; 67: 935.

Chapter 6

Becker MH. The Lacrimal Drainage System. In: Gonzalez CE, Becker MH, Flanagan JC. *Diagnostic Imaging in Ophthalmology*. New York: Springer-Verlag, 1986.

Duke-Elder S, MacFaul PA. The Ocular Adnexa. In: Duke-Elder S. *System of Ophthalmology*, Vol XIII. St Louis: CV Mosby, 1974.

Hamano H, Hori M, Hamano T, Mitsunaga S, Maeshima J, Kojima S, Kawabe H, Hamano T. *A New Method for Measuring Tears*. CLAOJ 1983; 9: 281-289.

Jones LT. The Lacrimal Secretory System and its Treatment. *Amer J. Ophthalmol* 1966; 62: 47.

Chapter 7

Duke-Elder S. *Textbook of Ophthalmology*, Vol II. St Louis: CV Mosby, 1938.

Schmidt TAF. On Slit-lamp Microscopy. *Doc Ophthalmol* 1975; 39: 117-153.

Chapter 8

Leibowitz HM, ed. *Corneal Disorders, Clinical Diagnosis and Management*, Chapter 15. Philadelphia: WB Saunders, 1984.

Sherrard ES, Buckley RJ. Clinical Specular Microscopy of the Corneal Endothelium. *Trans Ophthalmol Soc UK* 1981; 101, 156.

Chapter 9

Anderson DR. *Perimetry With and Without Automation*, 2nd ed. St Louis: CV Mosby, 1987.

Centers for Disease Control. Recommendations for Preventing Possible Transmission of Human T-Lymphotropic Virus Type III/Lymphadenopathy-Associated Virus from Tears. *MMWR* 1985; 34: 533-34.

Harrington DO. *The Visual Fields*. 5th ed. St Louis: CV Mosby, 1981.

Kolker AE, Hetherington J. Becker-Shaffer's *Diagnosis and Therapy of the Glaucomas*, 5th ed. St Louis: CV Mosby, 1983.

Nagington J, Sutehall GM, Whipp P. Tonometer disinfection and viruses. *Br J Ophthalmol* 1983; 67: 674-676.

Trobe JD, Glaser JS. *The Visual Fields Manual*. Gainesville Florida: Triad Publishing Company, 1983.

Chapter 10

Behrendt T. Fluorescein Angiography. In: Duane TD, ed. *Clinical Ophthalmology*, Vol 3, Chapter 4. Phildelphia: Harper & Row, 1983.

Behrendt T. Ophthalmoscopy and the Normal Fundus. In: Duane TD, ed. *Clinical Ophthalmology*, Vol 3, Chapter 3. Philadelphia: Harper & Row, 1983.

McLeod D, Hillman J, Restori M. Ultrasound. *Trans Ophthalmol Soc UK* 1981; 101: 137.

Schmidt TAF. On slit-lamp microscopy. *Doc Ophthal* 1975; 39: 117-153.

Weigelin E, Lobstein A. *Ophthalmodynamometry*. New York: Hafner Publishing Company, 1963.

Chapter 11

Gonzalez FC, Becker MH, Flanagan JC. *Diagnostic Imaging in Ophthalmology*. New York: Springer-Verlag, 1987.

Chapter 12

Davson H. *The Physiology of the Eye*, 3rd ed. New York: Academic Press Inc., 1972.

Duane TD, ed. *Clinical Ophthalmology*, Vol 1, Refraction. Hagerstown MD: Harper and Row, 1983.

Duke-Elder S. *Practice of Refraction*, 9th ed. Edinburgh: Churchill Livingstone, 1978.

Halliday BL. Calculation of Intraocular Lens Power—Results in Practice. *Trans Ophthalmol Soc UK* 1986; 105: 435.

Chapter 13

Anonymous. Temporal Artery Biopsy (Editorial). *Lancet* 1983; 1: 396-397.

Index

Altitudinal field defects 20, 22-23
Amblyopia 8
Ametropia, high 120
Amsler chart 118
Angiography, fluorescein 43, 136-140
Anterior chamber 88-90
Anterior chiasmal syndrome 109
Applanation tonometry
 Goldmann 91-97
 Perkins 97
Arteritis giant cell 167
Astigmatism 120, 132, 154
Atropine, systemic 15
Autofluorescence 140

Behçet's disease 139
Benoxinate hydrochloride 4%, 93
Best's disease 49
Bielschowsky head tilt test 31
Binocular vision 59
Biometry 162-164
Bjerrum (tangent) screen 98-100
Blind spot 107

Cataracts 9, 111, 134
Children, examining 7, 15
Chloroquine 111
Colour vision 16-19
Computerized tomography (CT) 43, 45-47, 143-144
Conjunctiva
 scraping 82
 swab 81
Contact lenses, diagnostic 129-132
Contrast sensitivity 14
Cornea
 Fuch's dystrophy 87
 pachymetry 88-90
 reflex 38
 scraping 83-84
 specular microscopy 86-87
 ulcers
  scraping 83
  staining 79, 80
Cotton thread tear measurement 66

Cover test, alternate 55-56
Cover-uncover test 53-54

Dacrocystography (DCG) 66, 68-70
Diabetes 165
Duane's syndrome 33
Duochrome 156
Dysthyroid eye disease 47

E chart 12
Electro-oculogram (EOG) 48
Electrodiagnosis 48-52
Electroretinogram (ERG) 49-51
Exophthalmometry 40-42
Eye movements
 infranuclear disorders 26-33
 pursuit 33
 saccades 33-35
 supranuclear disorders 33-35

Fixation 58
Fluorescein
 angiography 136-139
 corneal ulcer stained by 79
 Seidel's test 141
 in tonometry 93
Focimeter 148
Forced duction test 42
Foreign body
 radiology 142-143
 ultrasonography 135
Four dioptre prism test 58
Friedmann analyser 110-111
Fuch's dystrophy 87
Fundus, fluorescein angiography 136-139
Fundus contact lens 132

Gaze pareses 29
Giemsa stain 82
Glaucoma
 gonioscopy 114-117
 open-angle 108, 113, 117
 tonometry 91-97
 visual field testing 98-113
Goldmann 3-mirror lens 129-131

Goldmann gonioscopy lens 114
Goldmann tonometry 91-97
Goldmann-type perimetry 100-109
Gonioscopy
 in children 15
 for glaucoma 114-117
Gram stain 81, 83, 85

Hemianopia 20, 22-23
Hess charts 61-63
Hruby lens 126-127, 132
Hyperfluorescence 140
Hypertension 165
Hypofluorescence 140

Immunofluorescence 83
Infants
 binocular vision 59
 examining 15
 testing visual acuity 6-8
Intercanthal distance 40-41
Intra-ocular pressure measurement, see Tonometry
Iris dialysis 76, 117
Ishihara test plates 16-19

Jones' basic secretion test 66
Jones' primary dye test 66, 71

Keratometry 160-162
Ketamine hydrochloride 15
Koeppe lens 114

Lacrimal function 64-71
Lenses
 focimeter 148
 neutralization of 145-148
 see also Refraction and specific lenses
Levator muscle function 37
Lid measurements 36-37

Macula
 cystoid macular oedema 139
 disease, and colour vision 18
 function, Friedmann analyser 111

174

ophthalmoscopy 119, 124
Maddox rod 159
Maddox wing 160
Magnetic resonance imaging (MRI) 43, 47
Major amblyoscope (synoptophore) 60
Microbiology 81-85
Microscopy, specular 86-87
Myopia
  duochrome 156
  high
    colour vision 19
    fundus contact lens 132
    visual acuity tests 9, 13

Near vision 13
Nerve palsies
  Hess charts 61-62
  IIIrd 26, 30, 33
  IVth 31, 33
  VIth 32, 61
Neuritis, retrobulbar 52
Neuro-ophthalmology
  colour vision 16-19
  corneal reflex 38
  electrodiagnosis 48-52
  eye movements 26-35
  lid measurements 36-37
  orbital examination 39-42
  pupils 23-25
  radiology 43-47
  visual fields 20-23
Neutralization of lenses 145-147
Nystagmus
  congenital 13
  optokinetic 6, 33

Occlusion tests 7, 10-11
Ocular injury tests 141-144
Ophthalmodynamometry 132
Ophthalmoplegia, internuclear 35
Ophthalmoscopy
  direct 119-120
  indirect 121-124
  peripheral examination 125
  retinal drawing 124
  scleral depression 126
Optic disc
  diabetic neovascularization 120
  ophthalmoscopy 119, 124

Optic nerve disease 14
  colour vision 16, 18-19
Optics, basic tests 145-164
Orbit 29
  blowout fracture 63, 144
  cavernous haemangioma 135
  examination 39-42
Orbital granuloma (pseudotumour) 33

Pachymetry 88-90
Panfundoscope 129, 132
Parinaud's syndrome 29
Pelli-Robson letter sensitivity chart 14
Perimetry
  automated 112-113
  Friedmann analyser 110-111
  Goldmann-type 100-109
    background calibration 103-104
    procedure 105-107
    results 108-109
    stimulus calibration 101-103
Perkins tonometry 97
Phorias 158-160
Phoropter 156
Pituitary tumour 44, 46, 111
Posterior segment diagnosis
  Amsler chart 118
  fluorescein angiography 136-139
  ophthalmodynamometry 132
  ophthalmoscopy 119-126
  slit-lamp with accessory lenses 126-132
  ultrasonography 133-135
Presbyopia 13, 19
Prism cover test 57
Proptosis 39-42
  systemic tests 165
Pseudofluorescence 140
Ptosis 36, 37
Pupils
  relative afferent pupillary defect 23-25
  swinging flashlight test 23-25
Pursuit eye movements 33-35

Radiology 43-47, 142
Refraction
  centration 158
  cylinder axis and strength 154-155
  duochrome 156
  near vision 157
  phorias 158-160
  phoropter 156
  strength of sphere 153
  visual axes, separation 157
Relative afferent pupillary defect (RAPD) 23-25
Retina detachment, ultrasonography 134
Retinitis pigmentosa 51
Retinoscopy 149-153
  cycloplegic 153
  optics of 150-152
Rose bengal stain 80

Saccades 33-35
Schiotz tonometry 91
Schirmer test 64-65
Scotomas 20, 23
  Goldmann perimetry 107
  tangent screen 98
Seidel's test 141
Sheridan Gardner matching letter test 8
Slit-lamp (biomicroscope) 72-78
  posterior segment diagnosis with accessory lenses 126-132
Snellen letter chart 9, 11, 14
Squints
  accommodative 54
  alternate cover test 55
  assessment 29, 33
  binocular vision 59
  cover-uncover test 53-54
  fixation 58
  four dioptre prism test 58
  Hess charts 61-63
  latent (phorias) 158
  major amblyoscope (synoptophore) 60
  prism cover test 57
Stereograms 59
Swinging flashlight test 23-25
Synoptophore (major amblyoscope) 60
Syringing 66-68
Systemic diseases 165-169

175

Tangent (Bjerrum) screen 98-100
Tear film break up time 64
Tears 64-71
Temporal artery biopsy 167-169
Test charts 8-9, 12, 14, 16-19, 118
Thyrotoxicosis 33
Titmus test 59
Tonometry 15, 43
   applanation (Goldmann) 91-97
   digital 91
   disinfection of heads 91
   indentation (Schiotz) 91

Ultrasonography 133-135

Visual acuity tests 6-14
   1/60 (20/1200) or less 11
   adults 9-14
   contrast sensitivity 14
   infants, children 6-8
   less than 'hand movements' 12
   near (reading) vision 13
   pinhole correction 11
Visual axes, separation of (interpupillary distance) 157
Visual evoked potential (VEP) 51-52
Visual fields
   testing 98-113
   to confrontation 20-23
Vitreous detachment, ultrasonography 134

X-rays 43-44, 142-144

Zeiss four-mirror lens 114